Deeper into the Soul

Beyond Dementia and Alzheimer's Toward Forgetfulness Care

Nader Robert Shabahangi, Ph.D., and Bogna Szymkiewicz, Ph.D.

illustrations by Piotr Orlik

ELDERS ACADEMY PRESS

SAN FRANCISCO

Deeper into the Soul: Beyond Dementia and Alzheimer's Toward Forgetfulness Care, is sponsored by Pacific Institute and its AgeSong Senior Communities. This book is published by Elders Academy Press, a program of Pacific Institute.

The nonprofit corporation Pacific Institute would like to contribute to changing the mainstream view of aging. Rather than viewing aging as something to be avoided, we see it as an important phenomenon of life. Aging provides humans with the opportunity to mature and become elders in the true sense of the word: people of wisdom, rich in life experience, able to help us humans and our planet become more aware.

www.pacificinstitute.org

The goal of Elders Academy Press is to encourage people to value and embrace aging and to strive toward growing into the role of an elder.

Elders Academy Press
432 Ivy Street
San Francisco, California 94102
www.elderspress.org

First Edition

Printed in the United States
Distributed to the book trade by Baker&Taylor, New Leaf Distributing Company, and QP Distribution.

Interior design and illustrations: Piotr Orlik, www.studiop2.pl
Production artist: Emily Tanner
Editing: Bouyer Productions, Steve Boga, and Leslie K. Lewis

Library of Congress Cataloging-in-Publication Data

Shabahangi, Nader Robert, 1957–
Deeper into the Soul: Beyond Dementia and Alzheimer's: Toward Forgetfulness Care
Nader Robert Shabahangi & Bogna Szymkiewicz.—1st ed.
p.; cm.
Includes bibliographical references and index.
ISBN 978-0-9758744-8-6
1. Memory disorders in old age—Patients—Care. 2. Dementia—Patients—Care.
3. Alzheimer's disease—Patients—Care. I.
Szymkiewicz, Bogna, 1958- II. Title.
[DNLM: 1. Memory Disorders—therapy. 2. Aged. 3. Aging—
physiology. 4. Dementia—therapy. 5. Psychotherapy—methods. 6.
Social Support. WM 173.7 S524d 2007]
RC394.M46S43 2007
616.8'3—dc22

2007032317

Great human beings are those who do not lose their child's heart.

—Mencius

In Praise of Craziness, of a Certain Kind

On cold evenings
my grandmother,
with ownership of half her mind —
the other half having flown back to Bohemia —

spread newspapers over the porch floor
so, she said, the garden ants could crawl beneath,
as under a blanket, and keep warm,

and what shall I wish for, for myself,
but, being so struck by the lightning of years,
to be like her with what is left, that loving.

—Mary Oliver

This book is dedicated to you, the caregivers of this world. Thank you for your tireless dedication to service, thank you for the depth of your heart and soul–without you this world would be a very sad place, indeed.

Table of Contents

Foreword

If you have picked up this book, chances are you are either professionally involved with the elderly or dealing personally with someone who has lost the ability to remember. Or perhaps you are looking ahead at the frightening possibility that you may, one day, be among the forgetful.

Over four years ago, I watched helplessly as a wall suddenly descended in my husband's brain, cutting him off from his past and from the life we had shared for 35 years. Coping with this apparent catastrophe took all my attention and energy and it was a while before I could even begin to consider the future, and even longer before my curiosity and need would allow me to read.

Since that time I have reached out hungrily to everything that would help me understand what had happened to us. I've attended courses, visited care homes, started groups for elders suffering loss, and, most important of all, witnessed my husband coping with the reality of what had happened to his rich and creative mind.

When I first read *Deeper into the Soul* I almost wept with relief. Here is a book that speaks in one clear voice embodying all the voices I have sought in so many different directions. All the pieces of what I have been struggling to learn are here: information, understanding, communication skills, and, above all, a deep, encompassing wisdom to lift our experience from the mundane to the profound.

If you are a researcher, a hospital worker, a teacher, a caregiver, this book belongs on your desk or at your bedside. The creative, engaging format reflects the experience of the authors in teaching their philosophy and administering care homes. With each page leading the reader into an ordinary, recognizable question, they offer us four perspectives embodied and illustrated in characters who speak either from what they know or desperately wish to know. The Student-Intern asks our questions, the Psychologist offers us information, the Physician provides the science, and the Sage moves us above the obvious to the inspirational.

As I have learned, forgetfulness has many facets—physical, emotional, practical, spiritual—pushing everyone involved with it to search for something beyond simple survival. Every day is filled with challenge, whether you are dealing with someone you just met or your spouse of many years. When the man I love and know intimately asks me if I am his mother, when he forgets the way to the bathroom, when he doesn't know the day or the year or his age, I have to find something inside myself and him that will move us from this tragic winter into the land of warmth and possibility.

When we are with this forgetful person we may be asking why this long, seemingly empty, silence or this string of disconnected words, how to respond to him or her, or, most vitally, where to look inside ourselves for the peace and compassion we need to face and accept this mysterious other. *Deeper into the Soul* offers us a new perspective: clear, accessible, and inspiring.

When we wobble off-balance, shock-struck, we need something to hold us looking up, a life preserver thrown from above, and, under our feet, a magnet firmly embedded in the earth. This book manages to cradle us safely between the two.

Deeper into the Soul will push you further than you meant to go, surprising you into a smile of pleasure, a buzz of new learning, a challenge to your usual interpretation of meaning. Best of all, it will engage and enlarge your heart.

Elizabeth Bugental, Ph.D., MFT
Author of *AgeSong: Meditations for Our Later Years*

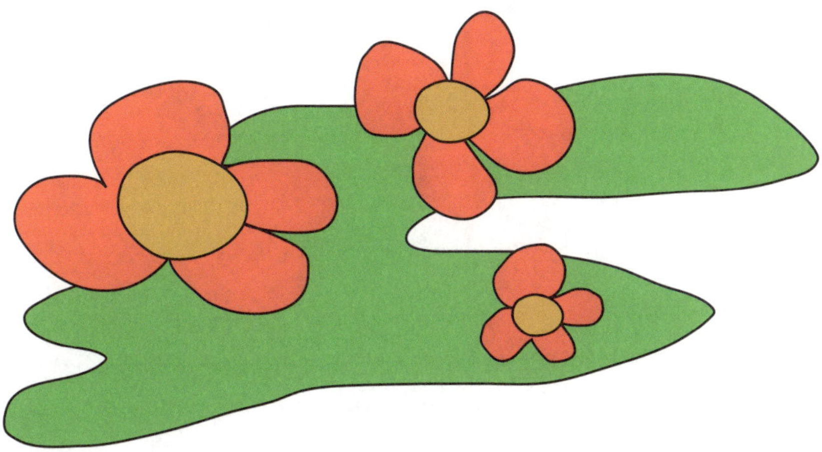

[F]rom ancient Egyptian to modern Eskimo, soul is a highly differentiated idea referring to a reality of great impact.

Anthropologists describe a condition among "primitive" peoples called "loss of soul."... Until he regains his soul he is not a true human. He is "not there." It is as if he had never been initiated, been given a name, come into real being.

Other words long associated with the word soul amplify it further: mind, spirit, heart, life, warmth, humanness, personality, individuality, intentionality, essence, innermost, purpose, emotion, quality, virtue, morality, sin, wisdom, death, God. A soul is said to be "troubled," "old," "disembodied," "immortal," "lost," "innocent," "inspired." Eyes are said to be "soulful," for the eyes are "the mirror of the soul"; but one can be "soulless" by showing no mercy...

— *James Hillman*

Acknowledgments

We would like to thank the individuals and organizations without whose help this project never would have been successful.

Our work is inspired by the work of Arnold and Amy Mindell, who first applied process-oriented techniques to communicate with people in comas; by our many students, interns, and volunteers at Pacific Institute, who keep sharing with us their amazing encounters with people with forgetfulness; by the work of Naomi Feil, who with her validation method pioneered a new approach to working with people with dementia; by the teaching of Max and Ellen Schupbach, who model for us how to work with awareness and have awareness work on us; and by the many elders living in our AgeSong Institute Senior Communities and elsewhere, whose love and care for us make this journey worth taking.

The need for a different manual for caregivers, one that would introduce a new, more respectful approach to people afflicted with what standard medicine calls dementia and Alzheimer's, was born from our work with the elderly in senior care facilities created by AgeSong and supported by the vision and work of Pacific Institute's gerontological and mental health programs.

Dr. Doris Bersing, the director of Pacific Institute, was a central, supportive force behind the work, and we greatly appreciate her passion for our project. Special thanks go to Elke Tekin, our brilliant sister, who was involved in planning the first draft of the manual; her commitment to a better life for our elderly remains an inspirational force driving our work.

A big thank you to Piotr Orlik for working with us throughout the whole process; his creative mind and talents were responsible for creating the graphics and cartoons in our book.

We are grateful to Steve Boga, whose editing eye and enthusiasm for both writing and the elderly helped us move the project forward, and to John Levy for looking at the manuscript and helping this book be more organized and structured.

Without the dedication and tireless work of our AgeSong Institute Senior Communities caregivers and staff, who inspired us with their gifts, this work would not have been possible. Appreciation also goes to Zen Hospice of San Francisco, whose approach to being with the dying so much mirrors our approach to forgetfulness here and to the Blue Mountain Center of Meditation, the work of Sri Eknath Easwaran, and to their many wonderful students, teachers and practitioners—their dedication to changing this world to a more loving, accepting and heartful place is exemplary and inspiring.

We are thankful to the Institute of Applied Social Sciences, University of Warsaw, and the Kosciuszko Foundation for helping us to organize research and teaching at the Pacific Institute and for supporting Polish-American cooperation.

We want to acknowledge the pioneers behind our different approach to communication with people in different states of consciousness: to Gary Reiss, Stan Tomandl, Ann Jacob, Tom Richards, Jan Webster, and Pierre Morin. We always stand on the shoulders of our mentors, elders, colleagues, and friends, who continue to guide us in our search for meaning and to open us to a wider range of human experiences.

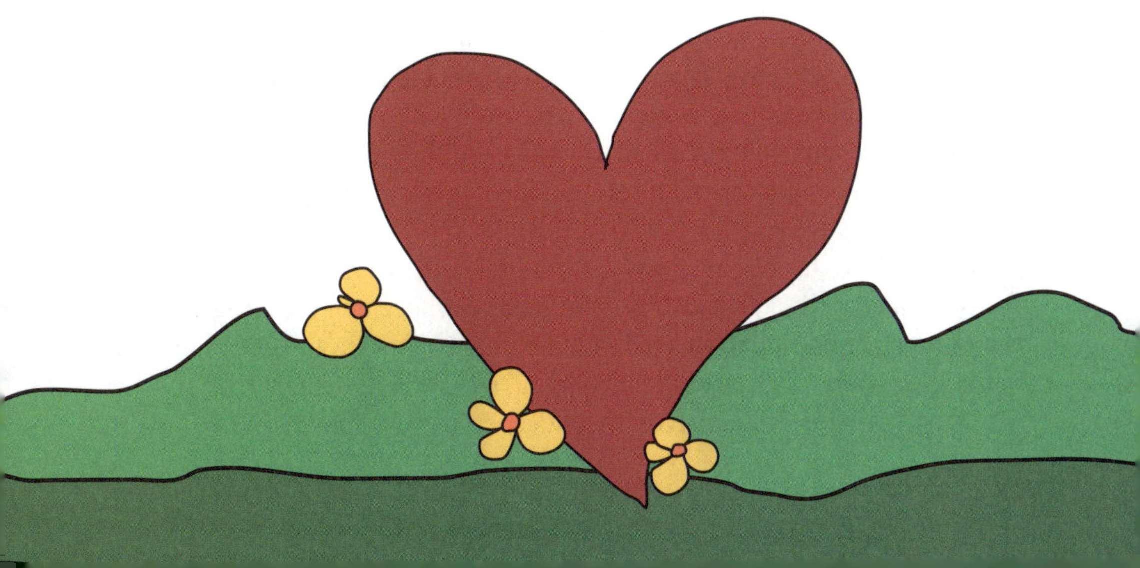

Introduction

Deeper into the soul—how do we do that anymore in today's busy, fast-paced world? We may enter into the richness of this question by asking: What is the meaning of our lives? Why are we here? For what do we live, do we struggle, do we mature? These are big questions seldom asked today. Yet these questions, and how each one of us tries to come to terms with them in our own lives, lie at the core of this book on entering deeper into our soul, on understanding more fully this phenomenon of forgetfulness.

To address the question of how we go deeper into the soul is to enter different terrain than we are used to walking in our everyday lives. Space and time begin to take on a new quality.

Case in point: one day we were waiting in our senior care home for a visitor and decided to sit next to one of our elderly residents. After acknowledging one another with small nods, we sat in silence on the small couch. Ten minutes later, the elderly man rose and said, "Thank you for sitting with me," then slowly walked away, pushing his walker ahead of him. Thank you for sitting with me. How simple—and how hard to do sometimes.

We would like to invite you to slow down for a moment and open your mind to the mystery of aging and forgetting.

Alzheimer's disease and other forms of dementia are a source of fear for many of us. We are afraid that we could lose the minds of our parents, relatives, and partners while their bodies are still with us. Moreover, we are jolted by the same fears every time we can't find our keys or remember the name of a friend. We seem to take it for granted that a meaningful life is possible only when one is blessed with excellent memory and cognitive abilities. From this point of view, life makes little sense for the millions of Americans and countless others around the world afflicted with forgetfulness.

In this book we highlight a basic attitudinal shift: Dementia is our teacher. Rather than simply a disease, dementia has purpose and meaning. Rather than being people simply in need of our care, people who forget can teach us about life and living. Rather than a burden, people with dementia offer us an opportunity to deepen ourselves, to go deeper into our souls.

This shift of attitude demands more than a slight adjustment in how we perceive the world; it requires a fundamental change in the way we look at ourselves and the world we inhabit. It requires foremost a curiosity, an openness to all that is. An attitude of *not-knowing* allows that which manifests itself in front of or within us to present itself in the way it *is*, not in the way we already know it.

This attitude demands a willingness to live in the question, to appreciate the mystery that envelops us. Our sense that we can control and direct our lives is only one possible truth. There's another possible truth, perhaps even more powerful, that places our direction in the hands of some other force, whether it be called God, Nature, the Tao, Quantum Wave, or some other word. From this point of view, events and relationships occur with meaning—that is, we ascribe meaning to them. As such, what happens to us, events we often categorize as good or bad, are part of our life-path, our destiny. The basic assumption here is that life has meaning, that somehow all—people, planet, universe—makes sense and has purpose.

In contrast, our prevailing attitude is less teleologically based and more grounded in a universe that is random. In such a universe we do not strive for meaning, but rather to manage the suffering that occurs when meaning eludes us. That is, symptom removal or alleviation is the final goal. After the symptom is removed, we don't need to understand it anymore. In a random universe we distinguish between good and bad, right and wrong, acceptable and unacceptable.

Those who believe in a meaningful universe suffer, too, but their suffering gives rise to a desire to understand the meaning of that suffering, to delve more deeply into the reason and purpose of the events that occur in our and other people's lives.

The first step in opening ourselves to the meaning of such events is to destigmatize terms that have come from a disease model grounded in the concept of a random universe. In the context of dementia, we suggest beginning by replacing the clinical term *dementia* with the concept of *forgetfulness*. In this way we focus on the experience of becoming forgetful and begin to understand forgetfulness as having a larger meaning and wisdom. The label *dementia* stigmatizes and dismisses the person with symptoms of forgetting. Although dementia has diverse and clinically challenging manifestations, we will emphasize forgetting as a central theme of this book, and call this phenomenon simply forgetfulness.

A person who enters forgetfulness loses what you and I have no difficulty remembering: our name, address, age, profession, and the like. Remembering such facts is certainly convenient, and a keen memory is often rewarded with appreciation, accolades, even money. Forgetting, in contrast, garners few positive responses and gets little respect. Yet it is a stage of life that so many humans go through. We have asked, "Is there a way to move beyond aversion, toward a collaborative experience of learning with the person who has become forgetful?" Our answer has become the content of this book and is partly informed by observing human interactions in an elderly care home. We often see strong reactions of family members and caregivers when someone with forgetfulness can't remember his or her or our names. Names are emotionally linked with identity. They differentiate us from others. Forgetting personal names is often a shock to those in contact with forgetful people. Clearly, the threat of losing our identity terrifies us.

But what is this phenomenon called identity? Is it who we say we are, or who others say we are? And we know how rich and complex we are as persons. When asked to identify ourselves, we often say: I am a man/woman, this young or old, live here or there, have this job, like this or that food, am with this or that person. Yet, we also know that it describes only a small part of us. When we are in an intimate relationship, we speak less of these demographic facts and focus on what is not so obvious: our dreams, desires, ambitions, vulnerabilities, and hopes.

Of course, these also form a part of who we are, the most important part, many would say. Thus, we see at least two aspects of how we define our identity. The first involves our consensus, factual reality. The other is more personal and involves our subjective, inner life.

This is not the place to enter into the rich topic of exploring the nature of human identity. Rather, we simply want to point out how malleable this concept of identity is and how it may only partially be related to our ability to remember. We suggest here that certain parts of our identity might even benefit from forgetting. Forgetting may allow for other, deeper parts of our identity to come to the foreground, parts our remembering keeps forgetting. The stories behind identity, behind remembering and forgetting, are not fixed but fluid; they depend much on our vantage point, our priorities, and our lives.

The medical definition of forgetfulness does not allow for any other possibility than the one it itself proposes: the person with forgetfulness is "less than normal," and hence nothing can be gained or learned from *demented* people. In contrast, if we try to understand forgetfulness from a different point of view, we will observe that as people forget and enter *Dreamland*, they can allow us to remember and capture that which is essential: to appreciate them for who they are and for what they show us from their place of forgetfulness. That is, if we do not make their world a disease, make their condition wrong, they can give us a chance to search for a deeper understanding of who we are, for our essential humanity. People with forgetfulness symptoms can allow us to be with what frightens many of us, namely staying open to the unknown, staying open to the flow and the unpredictable process of life.

This is not to diminish the pain and hardship both caregivers and those afflicted with forgetfulness can suffer. In fact, this proposed alternative view is meant to lessen the suffering and fear often associated with forgetfulness symptoms. It is also meant to broaden and deepen our understanding of human nature.

Forgetfulness can be understood as an invitation to remember something we may have forgotten in our hurried lives. Those suffering from forgetfulness—through their very forgetting—can remind us of the rich and complex essence of our humanity, an essence at least as much about being as about doing, as much about wonder as about knowing, as much about forgetting as about remembering.

Accounts of caregivers and spouses of people with forgetfulness tell us that their loved ones change as a result of this condition. They also tell us that their loved ones are still *there*, that a real person still lives inside. Perhaps people with forgetfulness symptoms are not present in the way that our consensus reality expects them to be, but they are there nonetheless. The story of an Australian psychiatrist further illustrates this point. One day he visited his parents—diagnosed as *demented*—at their house, where he spent some time exchanging basic pleasantries with them. As he was driving away, he sensed an urge to tell his parents about his relationship with a woman he had just met and the difficulties he was having with the relationship. He turned his car around, drove back, and reentered their house. Both parents were surprised by their son's quick return.

He told his parents about his new girlfriend, that it had been difficult to communicate with her and that he was confused about what to do next. The parents listened attentively to their son's story. After he'd finished, the father addressed his son in a reflective tone, saying that it would be best to tell his girlfriend his concerns and to have her do the same. This way they would gain clarity and openness and an understanding about each other's needs. The mother nodded in approval, adding that it would be wise to exchange these concerns as openly as possible, early in the relationship, so there would be no false expectations.

The psychiatrist, suddenly aware that he was talking to *demented people*, listened with astonishment to his parents' astute and wise suggestions. After he left his parents that night, he remained puzzled by their clarity, and wondered to what degree his attitude toward them influenced their behavior toward him. Was it his momentary openness to their world, his trust in their ability to *know* on a different level, which allowed them to connect to their son? Or was it just a chance encounter where, as the medicos would have it, the veil of the "disease" had lifted for a moment?

Another story comes from a nurse employed at an intensive care unit of a large European hospital:

During the usual morning rounds, a group of doctors, nurses, and students stood around the bed of a young boy in a coma. The doctor looked at the boy's chart and announced: "Well, nothing will come out of this one!" A moment later, the nurse saw a tear fall from the boy's eye. Others saw it too and they all stood in shocked silence. Later, the doctor said: "From now on nobody talks about the patients as if they were not present, no matter how unconscious they seem. We may discuss our opinions elsewhere. Perhaps that tear was just an automatic reflex, but the truth is—we don't know. Let's take it as a lesson in humility: what happens between body and soul is a complete mystery."

With the elderly, we are confronted with this mystery again and again. We so often experience deep moments of closeness with people who are supposedly not *here* anymore, who have problems with the simplest tasks of daily living. In this book we invite you to perceive contact with the forgetful elderly as an enriching journey for both sides. We draw from both modern science and spiritual traditions, all the better to understand this journey of forgetfulness and to make it more meaningful.

Being with forgetfulness indeed takes us deeper into the soul. Whether we experience forgetting in others or glimpse it in little moments within ourselves, forgetfulness offers us a gift, if only we are capable of seeing it as such. Perhaps loss is always a gateway to the real gains; perhaps we must forget in order to remember. In the words of Seng Ts'an who lived in China in the sixth century,

The great way has no impediments;
It does not pick or choose.
When you abandon attachment and aversion
You see it plainly.
Make a thousandth of an inch distinction,
Heaven and Earth Swing Apart.

For those who can truly lay aside their aversion or discomfort and learn to accept what is, the gifts of the soul await: equanimity, intimacy with the dream-world and its magical ways, slowing down to the speed of soul essence.

This book is meant as a practical guide for people who work and live with relatives or residents with symptoms of forgetfulness. It is also a guide for people who would like to shift their conceptual and emotional thinking, perhaps learning to make friends with their own forgetfulness. We offer tips and ideas for dealing with aggression or wandering, but we also explore new ways of understanding people for whom we care.

Completing this introduction, we would like to present four characters who will guide us through this book. They represent divergent types of knowledge, attitudes, and feelings, since contact with forgetfulness symptoms in the elderly evokes different emotions and thoughts in us. We see all these perspectives as important and valid.

Join our guides, as we search for meaning, comfort, clarity, and reason, on our journey deeper into the soul.

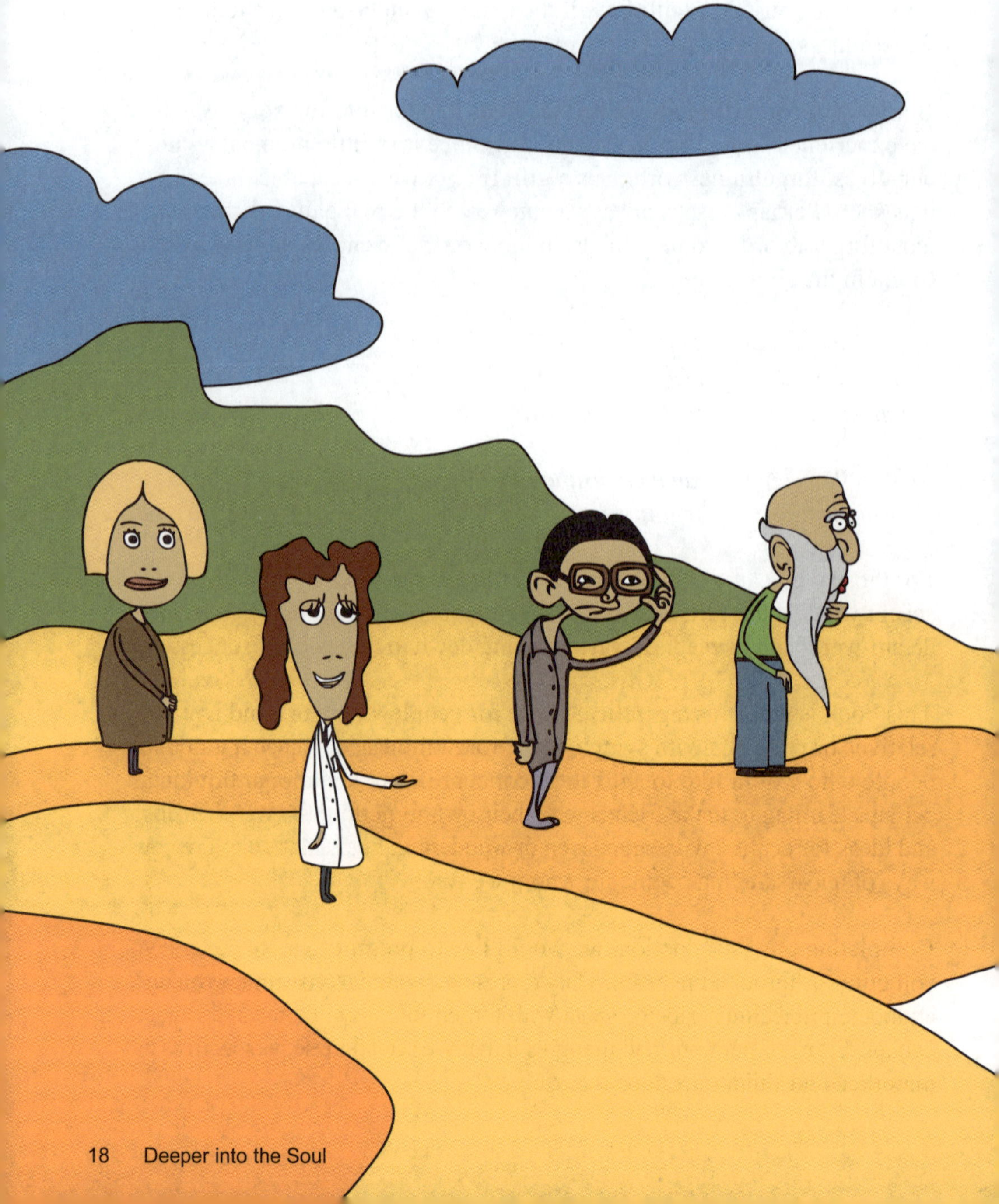

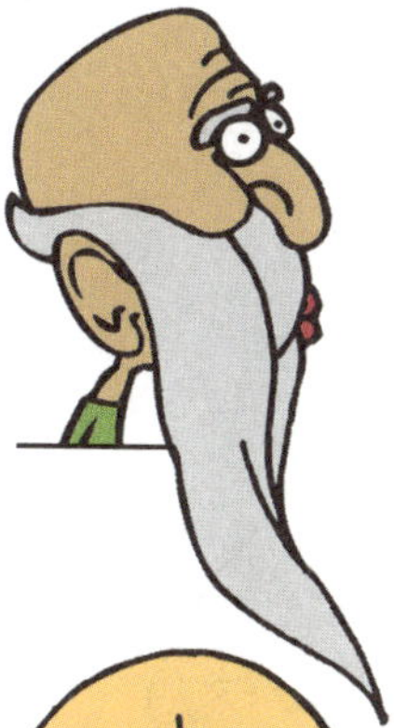

Master Susushi is a sage. It's difficult to pin down his tradition or religion, but we like listening to him. No matter how difficult or bizarre things are for our rational mind, he finds something important and meaningful there. He continually reminds us of the fundamental questions and mysteries of life.

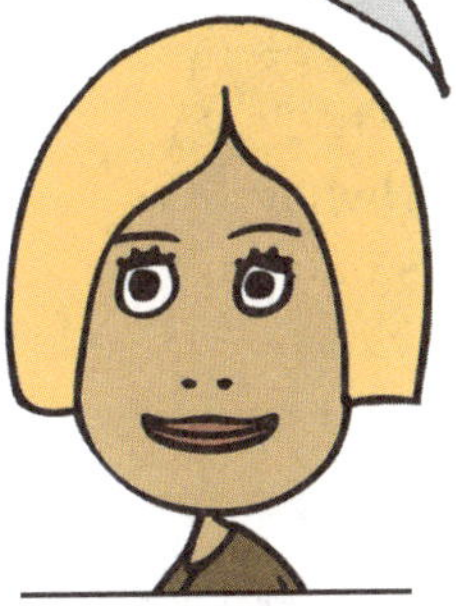

Ms. Jenny is a young trainee. She is enthusiastic but apprehensive. She has a clash of feelings when confronted with aging, erratic behavior, speech problems, and dying. She has deep questions about herself and her life; sometimes she wants to be comforted; but mostly she just wants to do a good job.

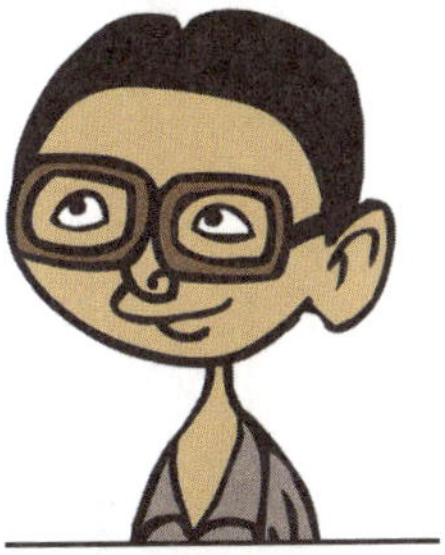

Dr. David has a degree in psychology and social work. He likes rational information, clarity, and structure. During his training, he wanted to learn how to understand and influence human behavior. He paid special attention to information that could be directly applied in practice.

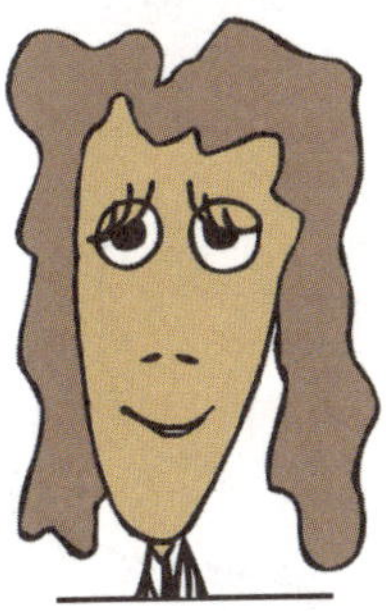

Dr. Karen is a passionate, competent physician and researcher. She loves talking about the brain and how it works. She will show us the amazing richness of the biological basis of our behavior. She will provide us with information about the medical understanding of dementia.

Sometimes these four people will talk to you directly; other times you will sense their perspective in the text.

Now we'll let them introduce themselves.

Sage
Master Susushi

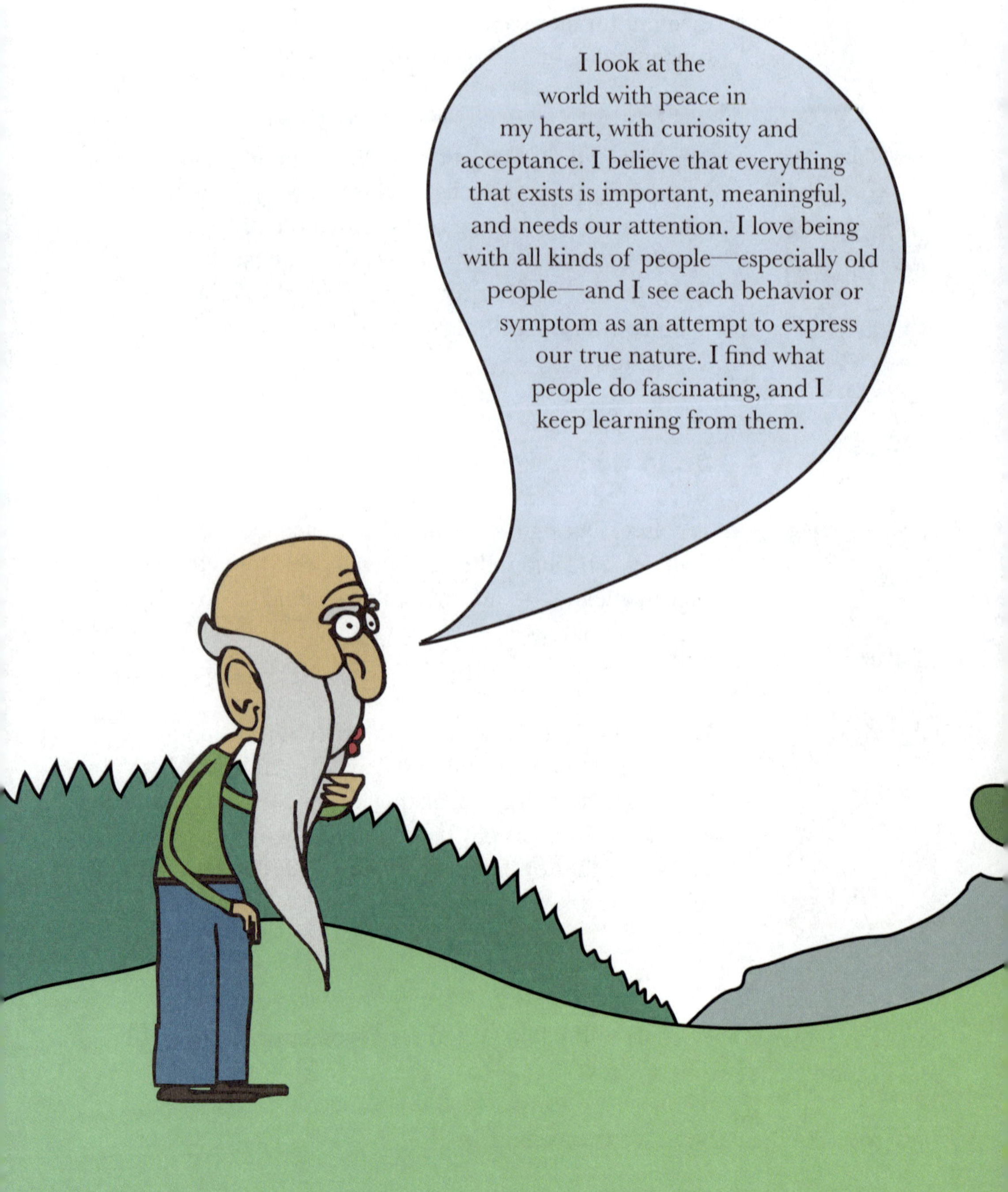
I look at the world with peace in my heart, with curiosity and acceptance. I believe that everything that exists is important, meaningful, and needs our attention. I love being with all kinds of people—especially old people—and I see each behavior or symptom as an attempt to express our true nature. I find what people do fascinating, and I keep learning from them.

Trainee
Ms. Jenny

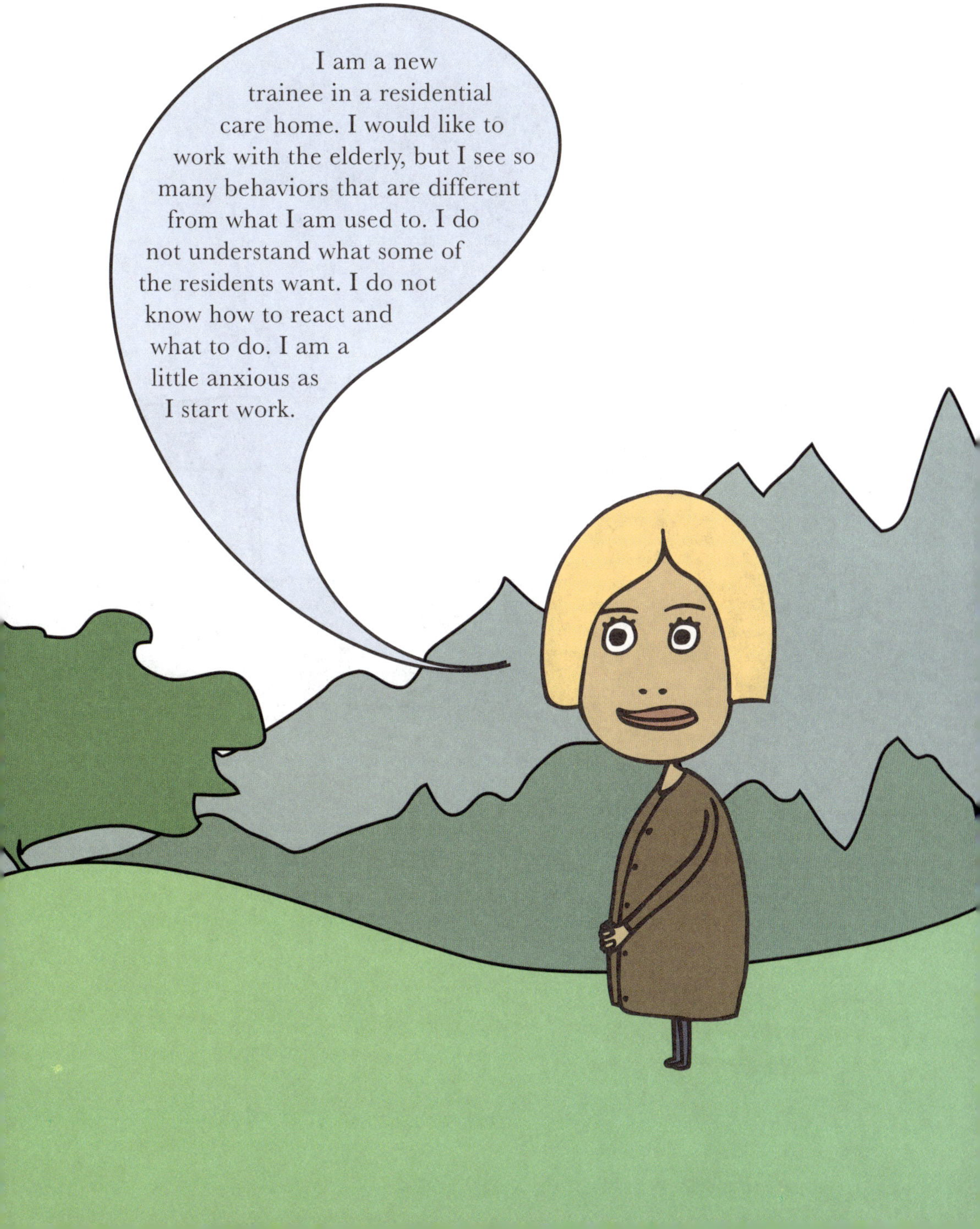
I am a new trainee in a residential care home. I would like to work with the elderly, but I see so many behaviors that are different from what I am used to. I do not understand what some of the residents want. I do not know how to react and what to do. I am a little anxious as I start work.

Psychologist and Social Worker
Dr. David

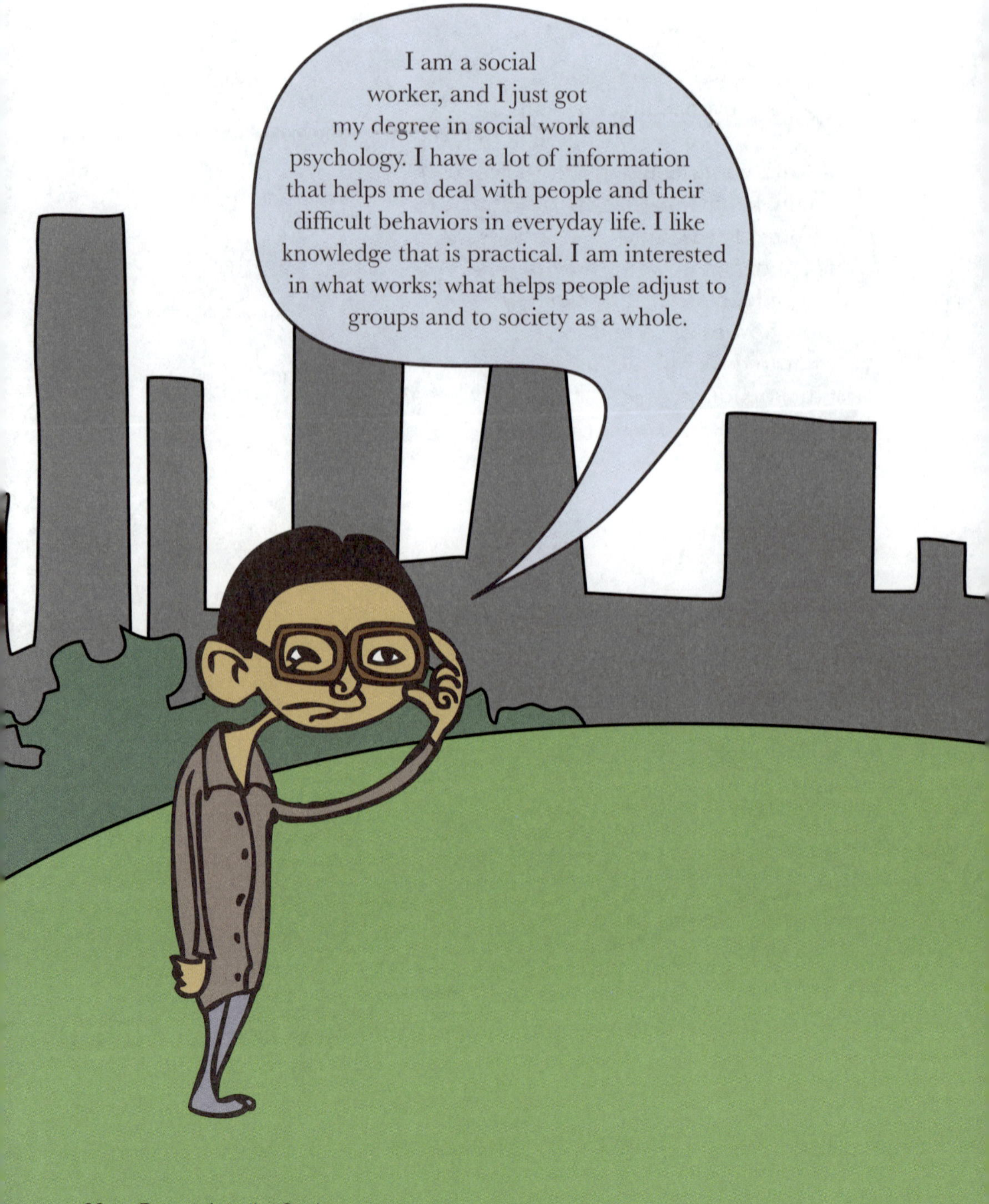
I am a social worker, and I just got my degree in social work and psychology. I have a lot of information that helps me deal with people and their difficult behaviors in everyday life. I like knowledge that is practical. I am interested in what works; what helps people adjust to groups and to society as a whole.

Physician and Researcher
Dr. Karen

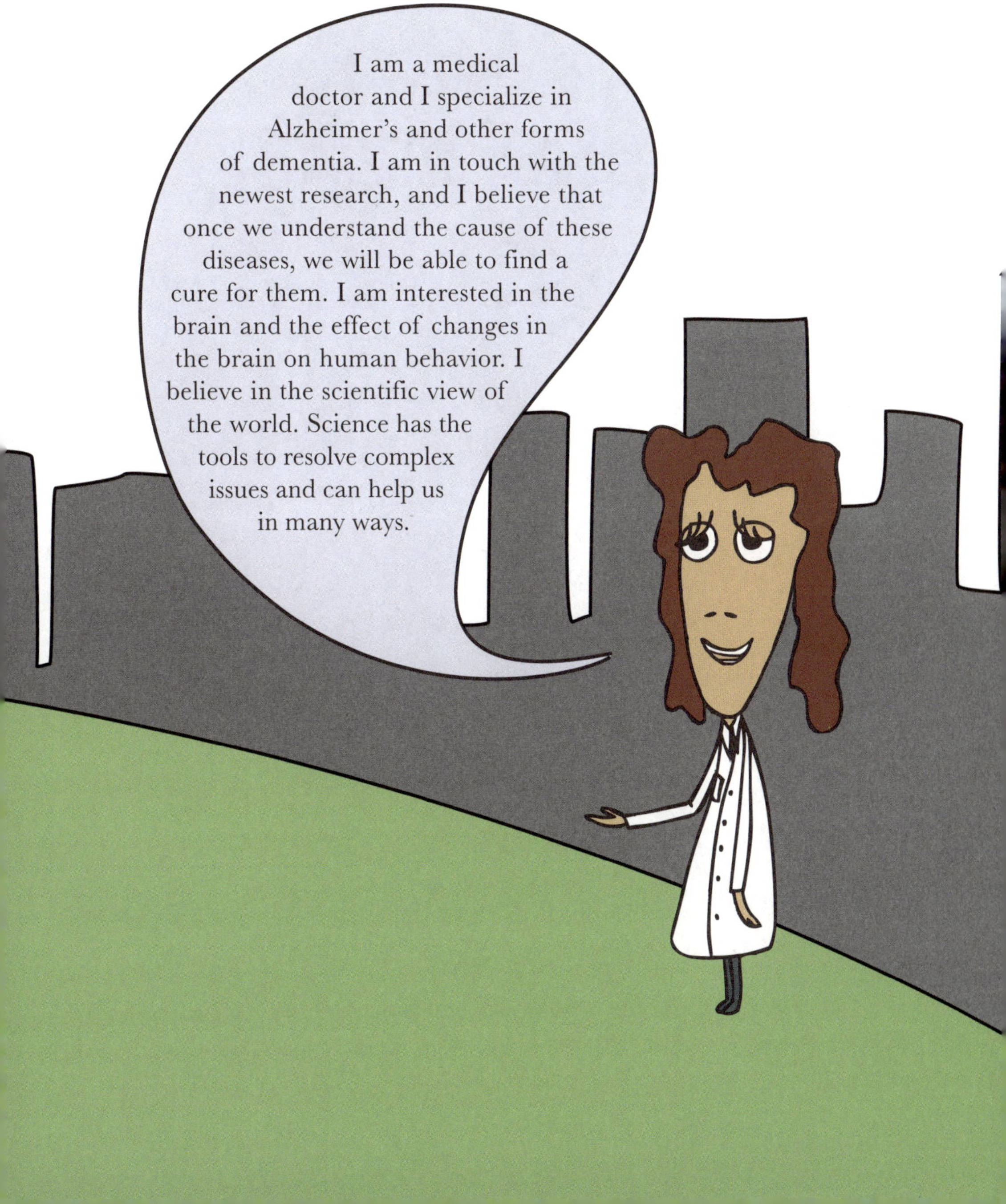
I am a medical doctor and I specialize in Alzheimer's and other forms of dementia. I am in touch with the newest research, and I believe that once we understand the cause of these diseases, we will be able to find a cure for them. I am interested in the brain and the effect of changes in the brain on human behavior. I believe in the scientific view of the world. Science has the tools to resolve complex issues and can help us in many ways.

Part One

Changing Attitudes

Genius... means little more than the faculty of perceiving in an inhabitual way.

— William James

Invitation

At the heart of our proposal lies a shift in how to understand and approach dementia, starting with the term itself. Rather than this often stigmatizing and demeaning label, we prefer "forgetfulness."

From a medical point of view, dementia is understood as a "progressive decline in mental functioning." It is caused by a disease or by damage to the brain. If we view the brain as the ultimate source of all psychic life, dementia seems to be a tragic loss of what is most human in a human being. With the loss of each brain cell, a part of the psyche disappears.

But are we sure that's true? Though the medical paradigm would have us believe that consciousness, or the psyche, is a product of the neurological activity of the brain, the mystery remains. We do not know where the soul dwells. We don't even know if it is the cause or effect of brain activity. We do not really know who is the boss, if there is a boss.

We want to create space for this mystery.

We see forgetfulness as a meaningful phenomenon, as a soul's search for itself independent of personal history or past memory. We do not know about the role of the brain in this journey. But we know from experience that everyone, no matter what their state of consciousness, is looking for contact with others and with his or her own inner experience.

In the first part of our book, we invite you to open up to this new attitude toward forgetfulness.

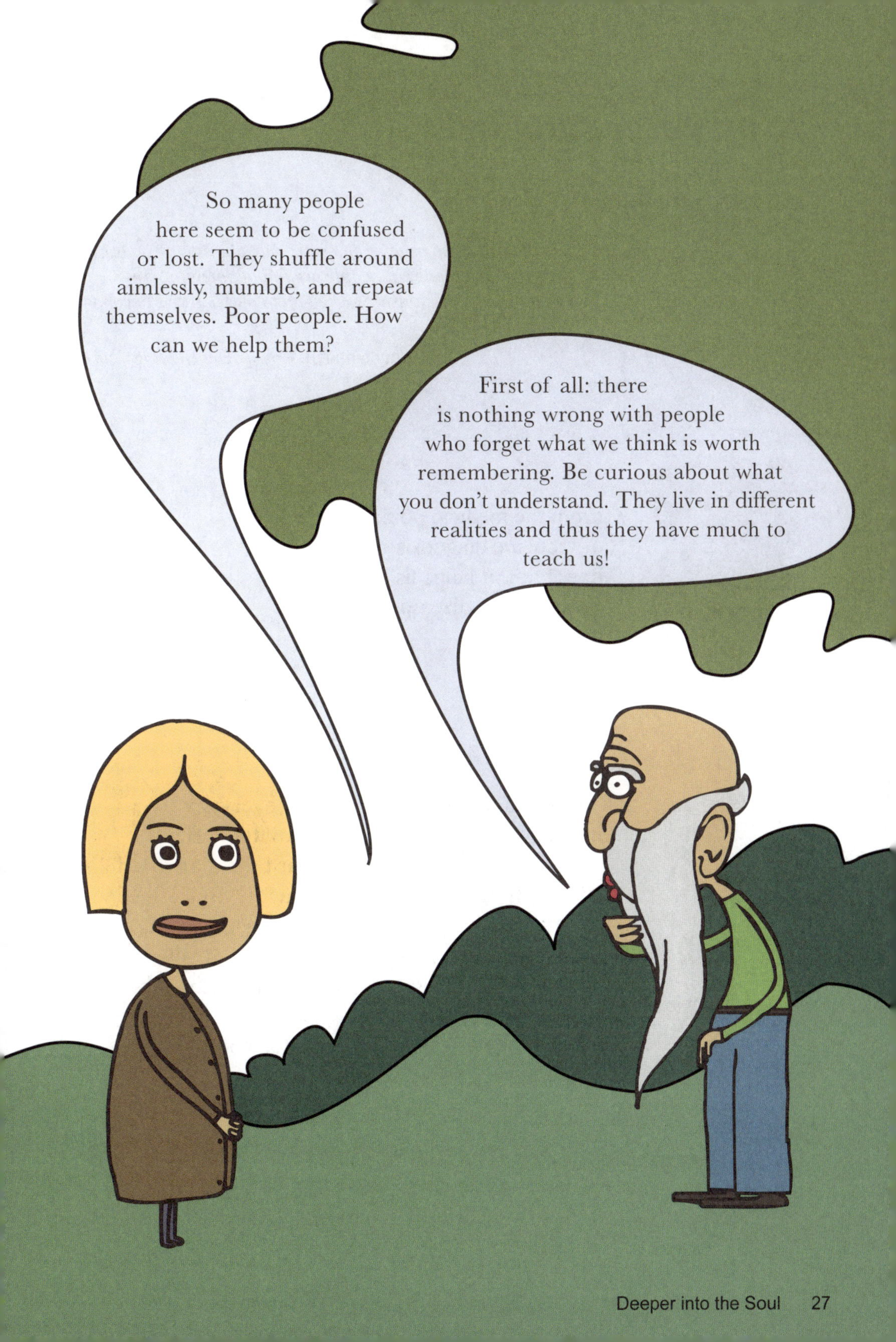
So many people here seem to be confused or lost. They shuffle around aimlessly, mumble, and repeat themselves. Poor people. How can we help them?
First of all: there is nothing wrong with people who forget what we think is worth remembering. Be curious about what you don't understand. They live in different realities and thus they have much to teach us!

Why *Forgetfulness*?

A New Approach

People do not operate as simply as machines that can break down and be repaired; people are full of potential growth in all states of consciousness–even up to and perhaps beyond the moment of death.

— Amy Mindell, *Coma: The Healing Journey*

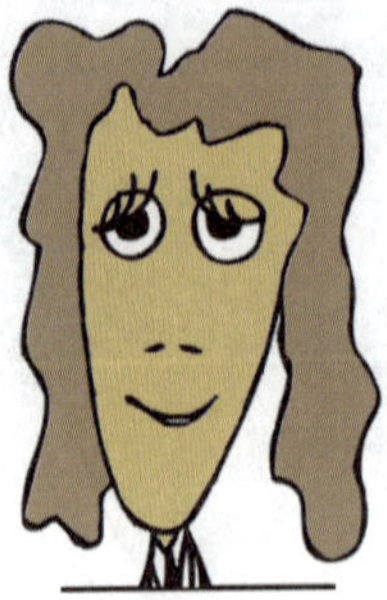

From the medical point of view the diagnosis is important. It helps us look for causes of the disease and find remedies.

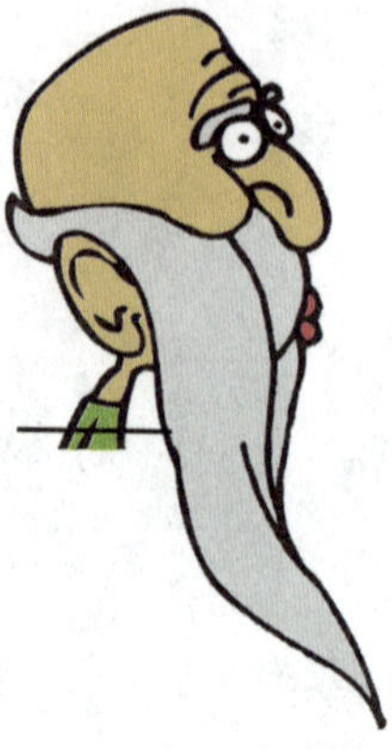

Yet the same diagnosis, used in everyday life, may become a label that immediately affects our emotions and attitude toward the diagnosed person. In the case of what is medically defined as dementia—a set of symptoms accompanying a variety of diseases—and especially its most common cause, Alzheimer's disease—the label sounds not only like a highly pejorative judgment, but also like a sentence: a person is going to become progressively "less" of a person.

We propose to make a shift, starting with a new concept of forgetfulness:

From Wrong to *Right*
There is nothing wrong with people who forget: they are going through an important phase of life and are trying to communicate their needs, feelings, and problems in their own ways.

From Disease to the Concept of *Meaningful Expression*
Symptoms disturb our normal behavior, our everyday identity, and often cause suffering. At the same time they carry important messages; our body talks to us in its own language.

From Directing and Controlling to *Serving and Learning*
As caregivers and helpers, we are here to understand and serve people with forgetfulness and to learn about our own future rather than to impose on them what we think is right.

Forgetfulness as Part of the Life Journey

Many spiritual traditions and areas of modern science have shown a great interest in various states of consciousness and levels of reality. Dreams, subjective feelings and visions, meditative states of consciousness, and even trances are no less important than the reality we ordinarily share. These states may give us access to the deep, meaningful experiences that are beyond our reach in "normal life."

As the symptoms of forgetfulness increase, a person becomes less and less present in our everyday reality. It can be frightening both for the disoriented one and for friends and relatives. But becoming open to various levels of reality can help reduce our anxiety and embolden us to look at forgetfulness from a new perspective.

Levels of Reality

According to Arnold Mindell and many spiritual traditions, we can talk about three levels of reality, or realms of perception:

Consensus Reality
This is our everyday reality: the world we agree upon, where we notice similar things and give them names. Consensus reality is considered the most "real" by most people. Here we agree on what exists and what does not; we share perceptions, even if our opinions and judgments differ. For example, we look at a table and agree that it is a table.

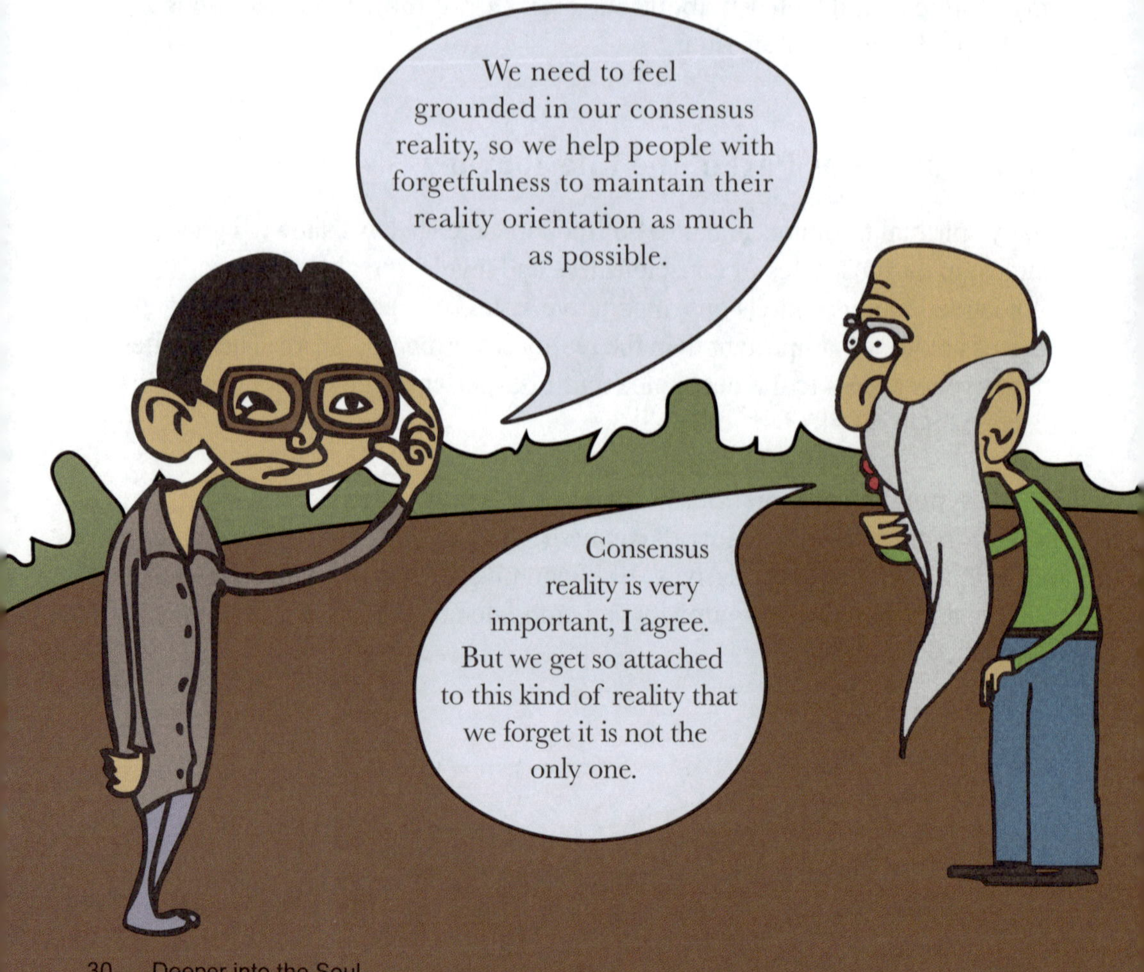
We need to feel grounded in our consensus reality, so we help people with forgetfulness to maintain their reality orientation as much as possible.
Consensus reality is very important, I agree. But we get so attached to this kind of reality that we forget it is not the only one.

Dreamland

This is the world we visit in our nightly dreams, visions, and other subjective experiences, such as emotions or pain. We see things that others cannot notice; we have feelings that are not easily explained to others. As Mindell puts it in his book *The Dreammaker's Apprentice:* "The parts of Dreamland are virtual; only you, the dreamer, see or feel or experience them. You cannot show them to anyone else. You can see your dream image, but no one else sees the same thing as long as their consciousness is focused solely on consensus reality." The table in my dream may be clear to me, but you don't see it in the same way. Yet, experiences in Dreamland are no less important than those from consensus reality. On the contrary, some of them are our deepest feelings and insights.

Essence

This is the root of all things, the oneness where everything is interconnected. Essence is the source of subtle tendencies that occur before they can be verbalized, such as a tendency to move before moving. Experiences here are the seed, or core, of an experience from which the other realms of consensus reality and Dreamland arise. Arnold Mindell talks about it in terms of energetic tendencies that dream everyday life to existence. Essence has many names, such as Great Spirit, God, Yahweh, Allah, Void, Quantum Wave function, and the Tao that cannot be spoken. Each person has a special, unique way of connecting to Essence. Sometimes it happens through deep altered states of consciousness. Coma, near-death experiences, certain meditations, as well as forgetfulness may open pathways to this Essence.

Levels of Reality and Forgetfulness

> *Without openness to our own altered states, we may have a tendency to marginalize people who do not fit into the communication norms of our culture. Hyperactive or withdrawn children, mentally challenged individuals, people in extreme psychotic states are looked upon as sick or disturbing. When we relegate people to such labels we never really learn to communicate outside a very narrow range.*
>
> —Amy Mindell, *Coma: The Healing Journey*

Our inner life, even when we are awake, has some dreamlike qualities, as, for example, when we "travel" to other realities. Think about the moments when your attention wanders; when you feel intense emotions, though other people cannot understand why; when you get as excited as a child or depressed and melancholic. Sometimes the same thoughts and emotions return again and again, recycling through our minds as if we were in a trance. Even while experiencing such states, most of us manage to stay in touch with consensus reality.

People with forgetfulness go to their inner world more often and in a more profound way than we do. They are afraid of losing contact with everyday reality, but they are also searching for something important in their own inner world. Their attention may dwell in Dreamland; they move inside of some stories rooted in the past and now going on in the land of fantasy. Sometimes they touch their spiritual core as they find their way to the Essence. As they try to find the meaning of their experience, they use movement, sounds, repeated phrases, or stories to try to communicate with us.

Attitudes

People with forgetfulness symptoms enter our world on different paths than those not considered to be forgetful. Behind the label of dementia we encounter people who are as sensitive and aware as anyone else. Granted, they try to communicate in a different language than the one we know. In order to understand this communication, we need to change our attitude. It helps to start with the following:

Openness

- Try to look at people without assumptions about what they "should" do, how they "should" behave.
- Treat people with forgetfulness as if they were your teachers: they will help you to slow down, to be more open and caring, and to get in touch with the essence of human nature.
- Keep learning to see, to listen, to feel with true compassion.

Curiosity

- Try to learn the meaning of each behavior and expression.
- Try to enable each person to share her feelings and experiences, no matter how different they seem from everyday reality.
- Remember that with each effort to understand the other, you expand your view of the world.

Acceptance

- Being confused, forgetful, or disoriented may be uncomfortable, but these are all natural states and none of them are "wrong."
- Each stage of forgetfulness is a meaningful part of the life journey, in which people go through important emotional and spiritual experiences.
- People deserve excellent physical, medical, and emotional care no matter how removed from our reality they seem.

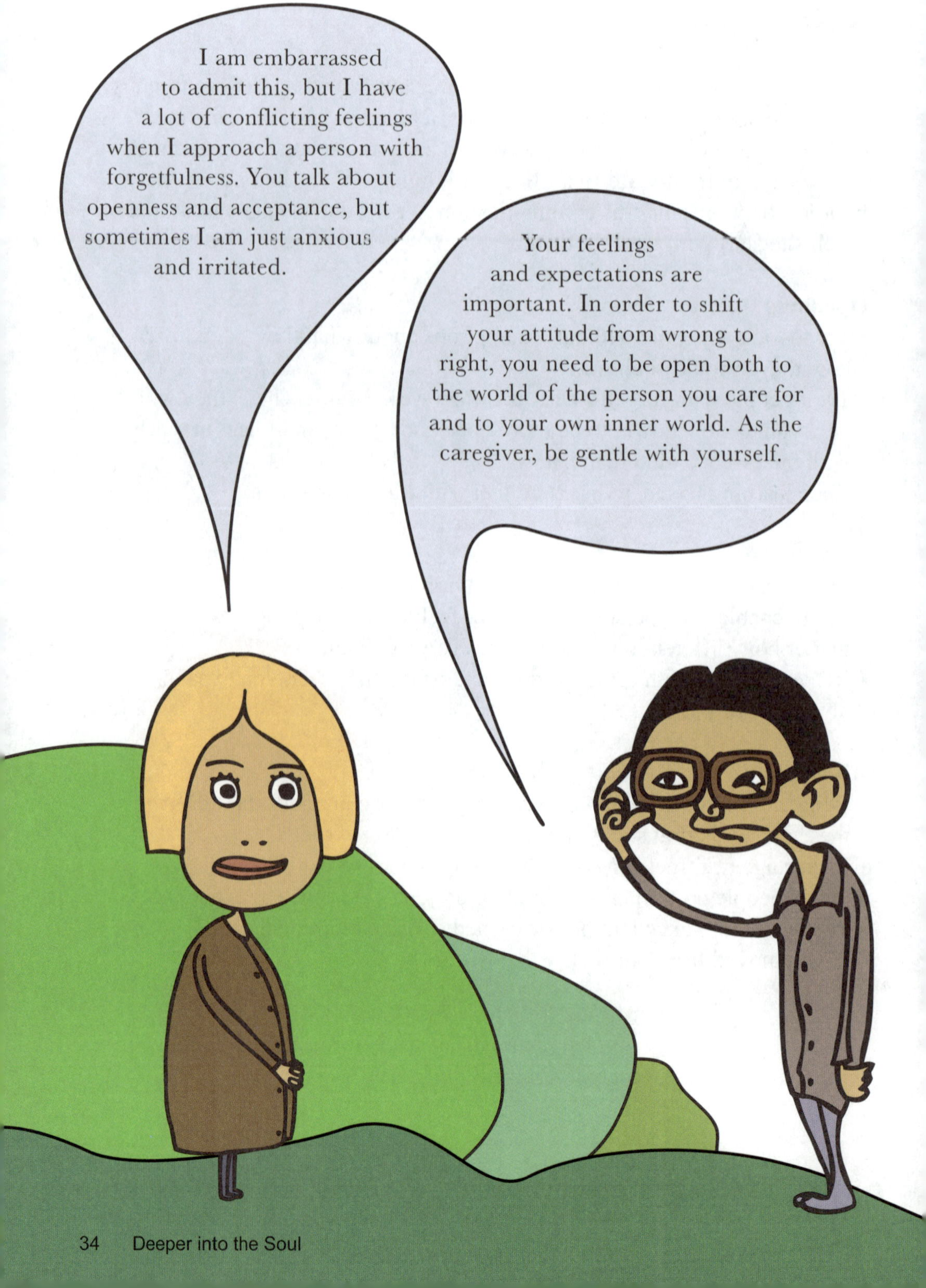
I am embarrassed to admit this, but I have a lot of conflicting feelings when I approach a person with forgetfulness. You talk about openness and acceptance, but sometimes I am just anxious and irritated.
Your feelings and expectations are important. In order to shift your attitude from wrong to right, you need to be open both to the world of the person you care for and to your own inner world. As the caregiver, be gentle with yourself.

Difficult Feelings

When we approach a person with forgetfulness symptoms, we often feel uneasy. Why?

- Our familiar ways of communicating and caring for others may not apply.
- We want to do our best, but often we do not know what that means for a person who is not quite *here*.
- Our own fears of aging, becoming dependent, sick, or dying get activated.

Expectations
We all have expectations about others. Many of us make the following assumptions:

- The person I feel close to will recognize me and respond to me in a predictable manner.
- *Normal* contact means that the other person understands me and responds to me verbally.
- The person I care for will appreciate now as well as in the future what I have done.
- The person will try to cooperate when I am helping her or him.

Though it is not easy, letting go of such expectations helps put us in deeper contact with anyone with forgetfulness symptoms. It is a process that requires attention, honesty, and support. When you try to give up your expectations of what is *normal*, different feelings will likely come up. For example:

- anger
- sadness
- helplessness
- confusion
- frustration
- pity

Make space for those feelings. Talk to friends and other caregivers; join a support group. To finally let go and make space for something else, you may need to discuss, rebel, mourn, and find a new way.

Dealing with Frustration

While being with a person with forgetfulness, you will sometimes experience frustration. It is a natural reaction.

Learn to Recognize Physical Warning Signs:

- Stomach cramps.
- Shortness of breath.
- Chest pain.
- Headache.

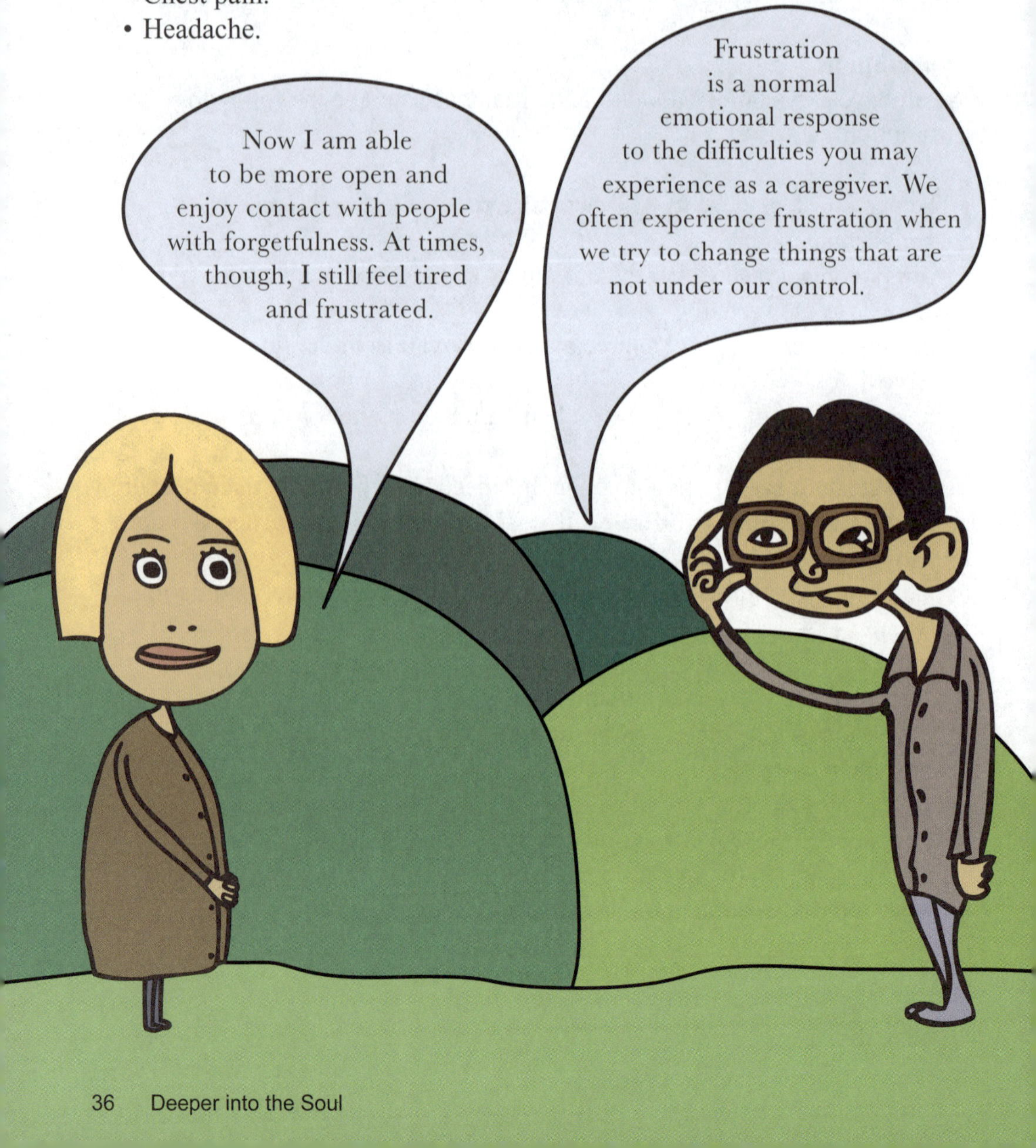
Now I am able to be more open and enjoy contact with people with forgetfulness. At times, though, I still feel tired and frustrated.
Frustration is a normal emotional response to the difficulties you may experience as a caregiver. We often experience frustration when we try to change things that are not under our control.

Find Your Own Techniques to Calm Down

- Count down from ten to one.
- Take a few deep breaths.
- Remove yourself from the situation (e.g., go to another room).
- Pray.

Long-Term Reactions

If you feel frustrated for longer periods of time, you may experience some of the following symptoms:

- Chronic fatigue.
- Anger at those who demand something.
- Irritability.
- Helplessness.
- Emotional outbursts.
- Weight gain or loss.
- Sleeplessness.
- Depression.

Learn to Take Care of Yourself

- Talk about your problems with other people, including your team members, friends, family, and support group.
- Adjust your expectations.
- Learn to ask for help and support.
- Care for yourself physically: eat well, exercise, and get enough sleep.
- Spend some good time with family and friends.
- Learn to express your feelings in a healthy way.
- Take time for your spiritual beliefs and practices.

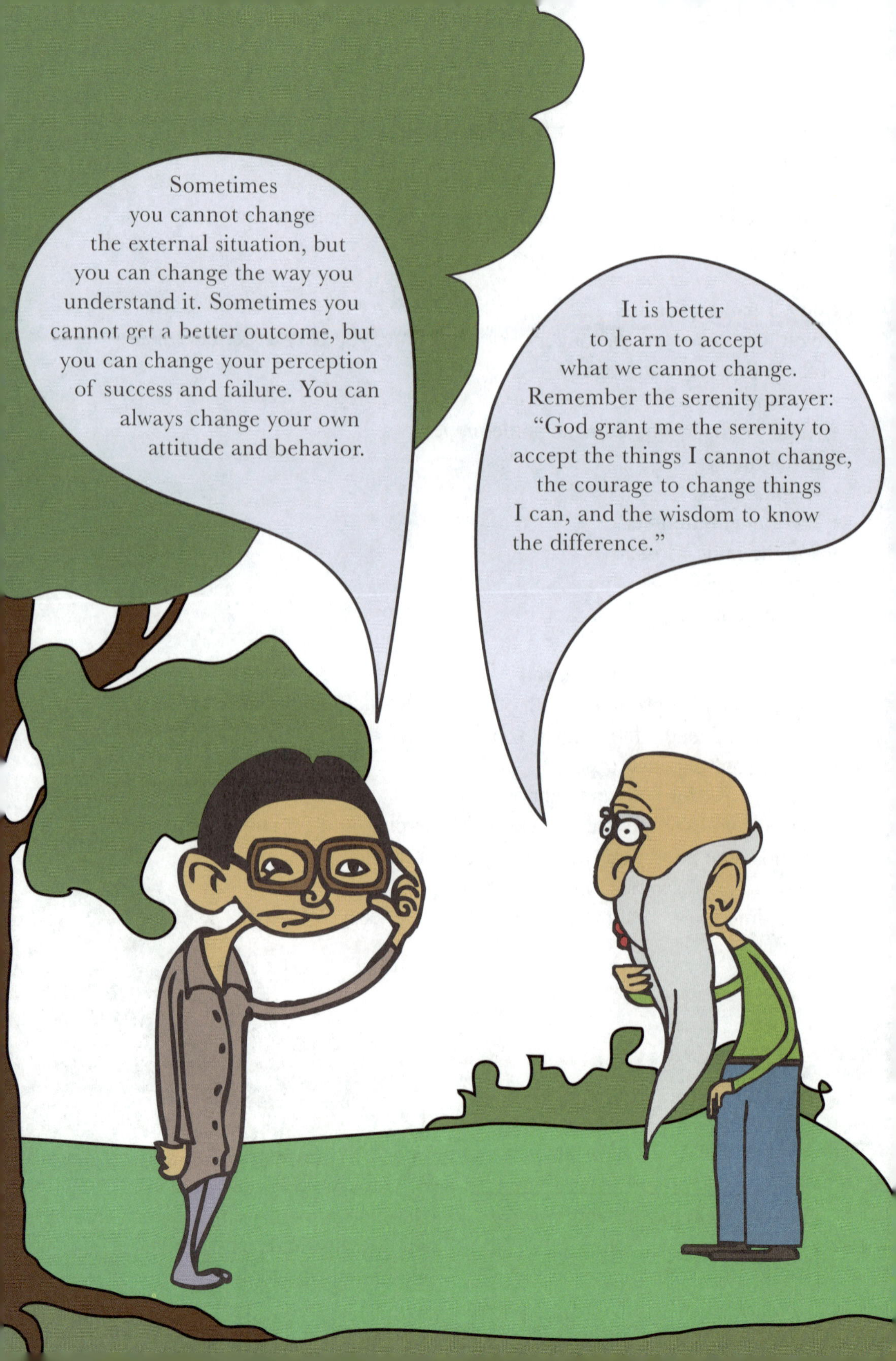
Sometimes you cannot change the external situation, but you can change the way you understand it. Sometimes you cannot get a better outcome, but you can change your perception of success and failure. You can always change your own attitude and behavior.
It is better to learn to accept what we cannot change. Remember the serenity prayer: "God grant me the serenity to accept the things I cannot change, the courage to change things I can, and the wisdom to know the difference."

Frustrating Versus Helpful Attitudes

Attitudes have a plethora of origins; some come from our basic assumptions and deep belief systems; others result from a traumatic event or life experience. Some of them are helpful while dealing with forgetfulness; others are a source of frustration. Compare the following:

Frustrating:	**Helpful**:
• Forgetting is wrong.	• Forgetting about this world helps put us in touch with our essential feelings, with our spiritual core.
• Alzheimer's is just a disease with no cure: it is the worst thing that can happen to you when you are old.	• Alzheimer's is a mystery: we move away from consensus reality into a realm of experiences that we don't yet understand.
• A person whose mental functioning deteriorates is less of a person.	• A person with forgetfulness who is disoriented and needs our help can teach us about the deepest human values: love, care, tolerance.
• People with forgetfulness are just a burden for their caregivers.	• We can enjoy the beauty of little moments together with someone who forgets.
• People with forgetfulness cannot do anything on their own: they experience only failures, no successes.	• We can always help a person use and enjoy remaining capabilities.
• We should ignore how people with forgetfulness change and expect them to act the way they used to.	• Any day may bring a change—we need to learn to go with the flow.
• People with forgetfulness are not able to communicate with us.	• We can learn different ways of communication if we remember that holding hands may be more important than words.

Join People Where They Are

Caring for a person with forgetfulness symptoms is like dancing between different worlds.

The World of Remembering

This is the world we know. It seems logical. We can learn, do things, achieve our goals, become mothers, fathers, workers, and heroes. We look forward to the future. We have orientation in time and space, and we share it with others. So many things seem obvious: we recognize objects, people, food, time of the day. We can take care of ourselves. We love, hate, enjoy, regret; all these feelings are part of our personal history.

The World of Forgetting

Things are not what they used to be. Words go away. Surroundings become unfamiliar. Sometimes it is scary. Who am I? What am I doing here? Some little islands of memory remain. On one island may be some treasure: the important issue that we overlooked before in our life. Feelings are intense, but it is difficult to understand them. Memories go away. We want them back! Or perhaps we don't need them anymore? We are going into the unknown, with little preparation or guidance. Sometimes we do not know how to make sense of our experience, though we feel it has great importance!

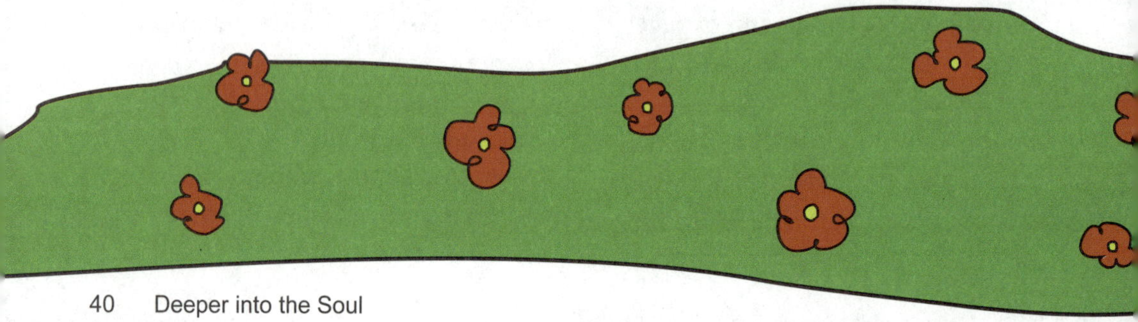

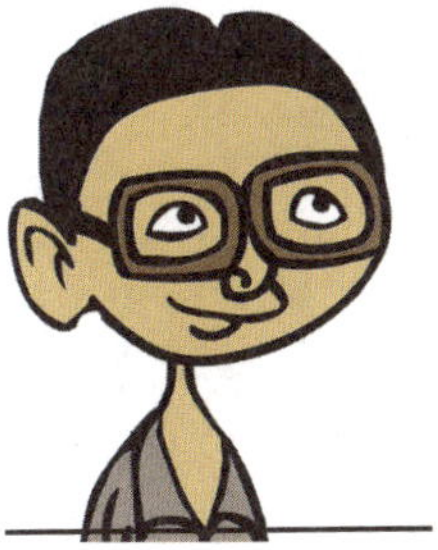

Think about what happens in consensus reality. People with forgetfulness symptoms in *our world* may often:

- Feel disoriented: the world around them becomes more and more incomprehensible.
- Experience disconcerting emotions: anxiety, anger, helplessness.
- Lose the ability to locate things in space.
- Have difficulty recognizing objects.
- Lose some ability to understand words and to use language.
- Try to find a way back to the everyday world after losing sight, hearing, memory, or mobility.
- Try to communicate through what remains—sound, movement, body, touch, gesture.

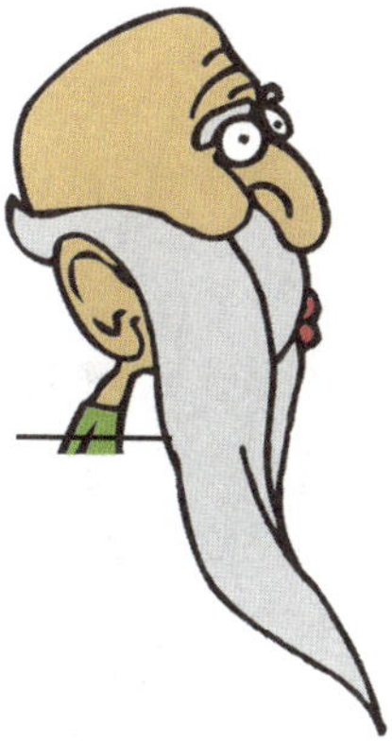

Think about what happens when a person with forgetfulness goes to the *other world*. This person often:

- Feels lonely.
- Looks for guidance.
- Urgently strives to understand his or her experiences.
- Needs to use time to complete unfinished past stories or to resolve relationship issues (using us and the surroundings as actors and objects in her inner drama).
- Needs to express present emotions as well as feelings previously unexpressed.
- Needs to be nurtured.
- Needs to be seen, understood, and validated.
- Needs to contact the center of self.
- Needs to find a way to his or her spiritual center (for some people, God).

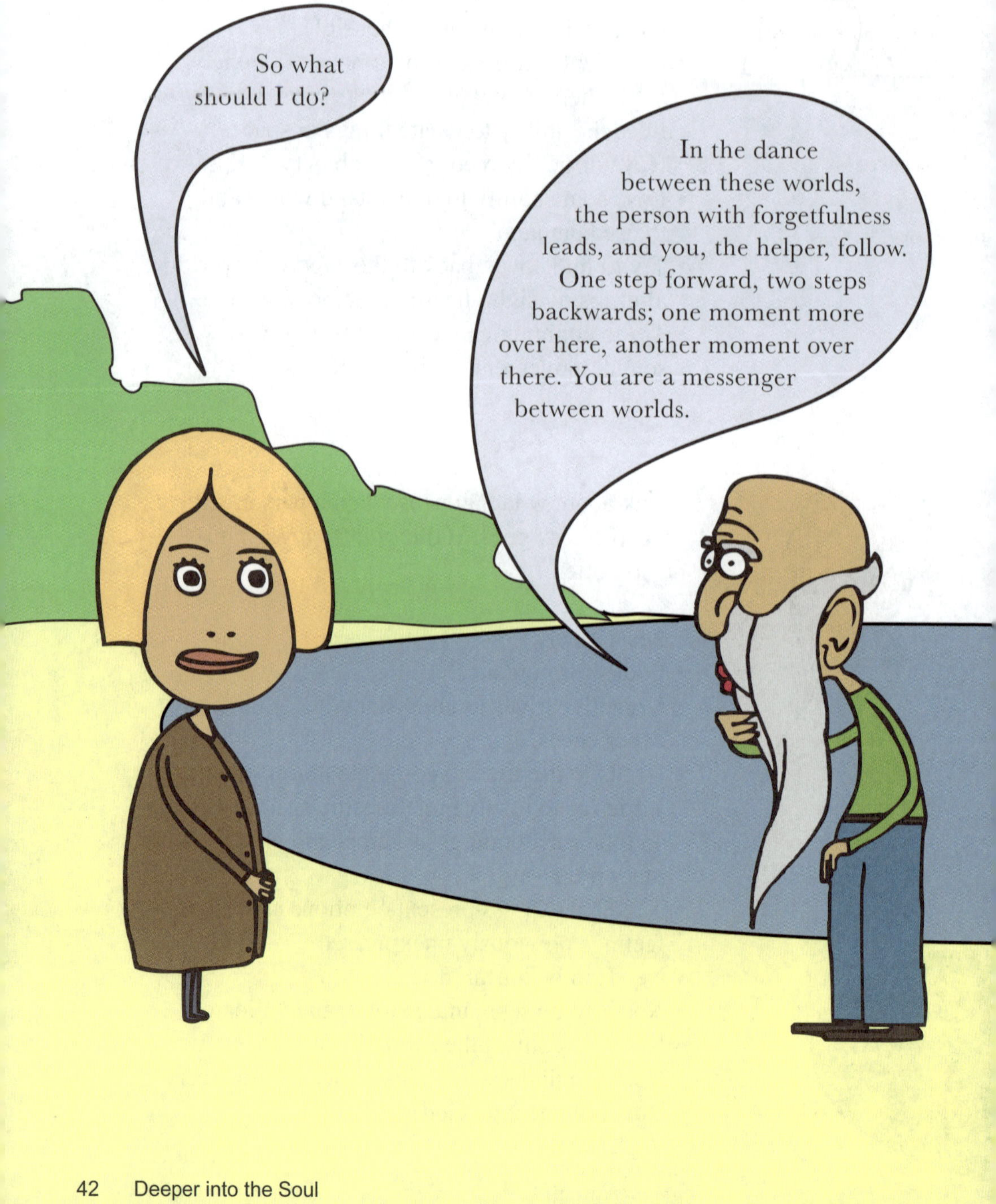

So what should I do?
In the dance between these worlds, the person with forgetfulness leads, and you, the helper, follow. One step forward, two steps backwards; one moment more over here, another moment over there. You are a messenger between worlds.

Toward the World of Remembering

- Help a person use existing capabilities.
- Enable little feelings of success every day.
- Engage in group activities.
- Create opportunities for deep social contacts.
- Support reliable daily routines.
- Encourage people to take part in memory training if they enjoy it.
- Help a person feel important every moment you are together.
- Help find identity through work from the past.

Toward the World of Forgetting

- Acknowledge the feelings of grief, sadness, and anger that arise as people begin to forget the reality of memory.
- Do not judge their behavior from your point of view.
- Try to learn as much as you can about their reality.
- Stay in contact with feelings, both yours and those of the forgetful person.
- Use the full spectrum of different ways of communication.

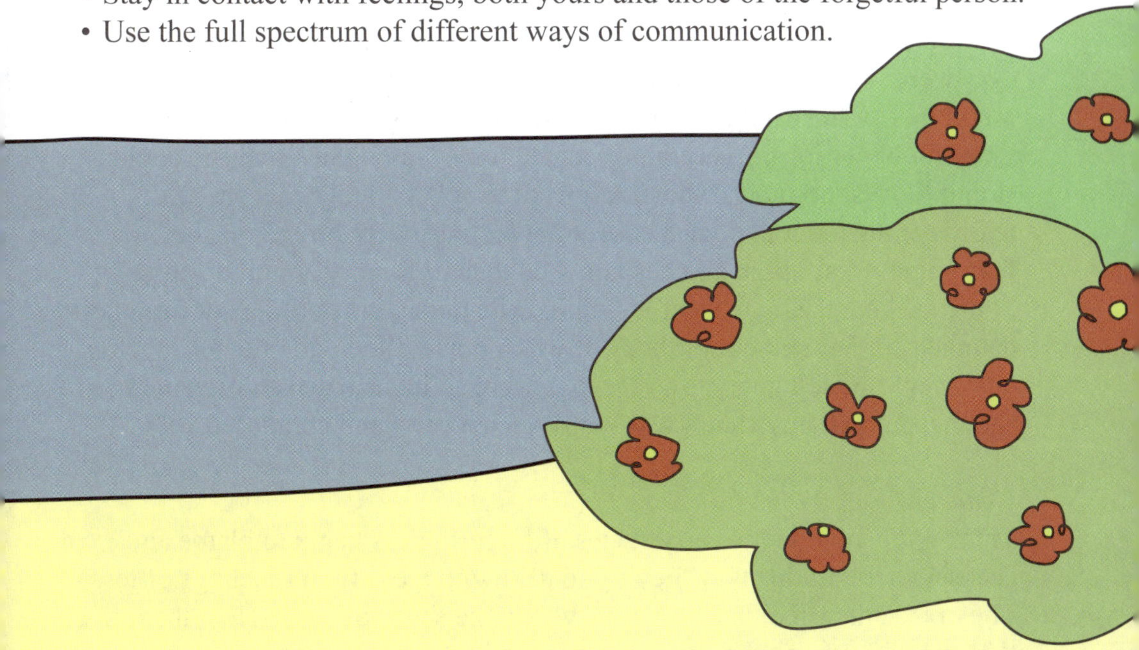

Symbolic Stories

> *Old people lose memory and surrender present-day factual thinking in order to heal old wounds from the past before they die.*
>
> —Naomi Feil, *The Validation Breakthrough*

How can we understand these *other realities* better? Imagine you are entering a fairy tale land. Words and stories have symbolic meaning; they speak about important feelings, even if facts or events are confused. If you allow yourself to enter this fantasy land, inside of the story you can meet a person with forgetfulness and to an extent understand her emotions, longings, and needs.

Consider the following stories:

Magical Purse

Suzan tried to stay calm and composed. She used to have her life under control. Then things began to change. She was in a care home now. Her eyes weren't serving her the way they used to. She lost her hearing and mobility. Her husband died, and her children and grandchildren moved away for better jobs. Everything seemed to be leaving her, and she couldn't stop it. It was too much. She didn't want to acknowledge that she was really getting older and weaker. But the feelings were boiling inside: fear, anger, frustration, and despair. And then, this story about the purse! Someone kept trying to steal it, her favorite purse, the one she got from her daughter for her sixtieth birthday. It was a purse filled with memories. How dare they! She felt angry. The feelings were so intense that she began to shout and cry, though she was usually such a calm and composed person.

Comment

Many old people in the early stages of forgetfulness begin to blame and accuse others. In this way they try to deal with the difficult feelings of loss. They place their feelings into a story to make sense of them. Help them tell their story. Even if the facts seem inaccurate to you, they have emotional truth. Remember, it is a magical purse!

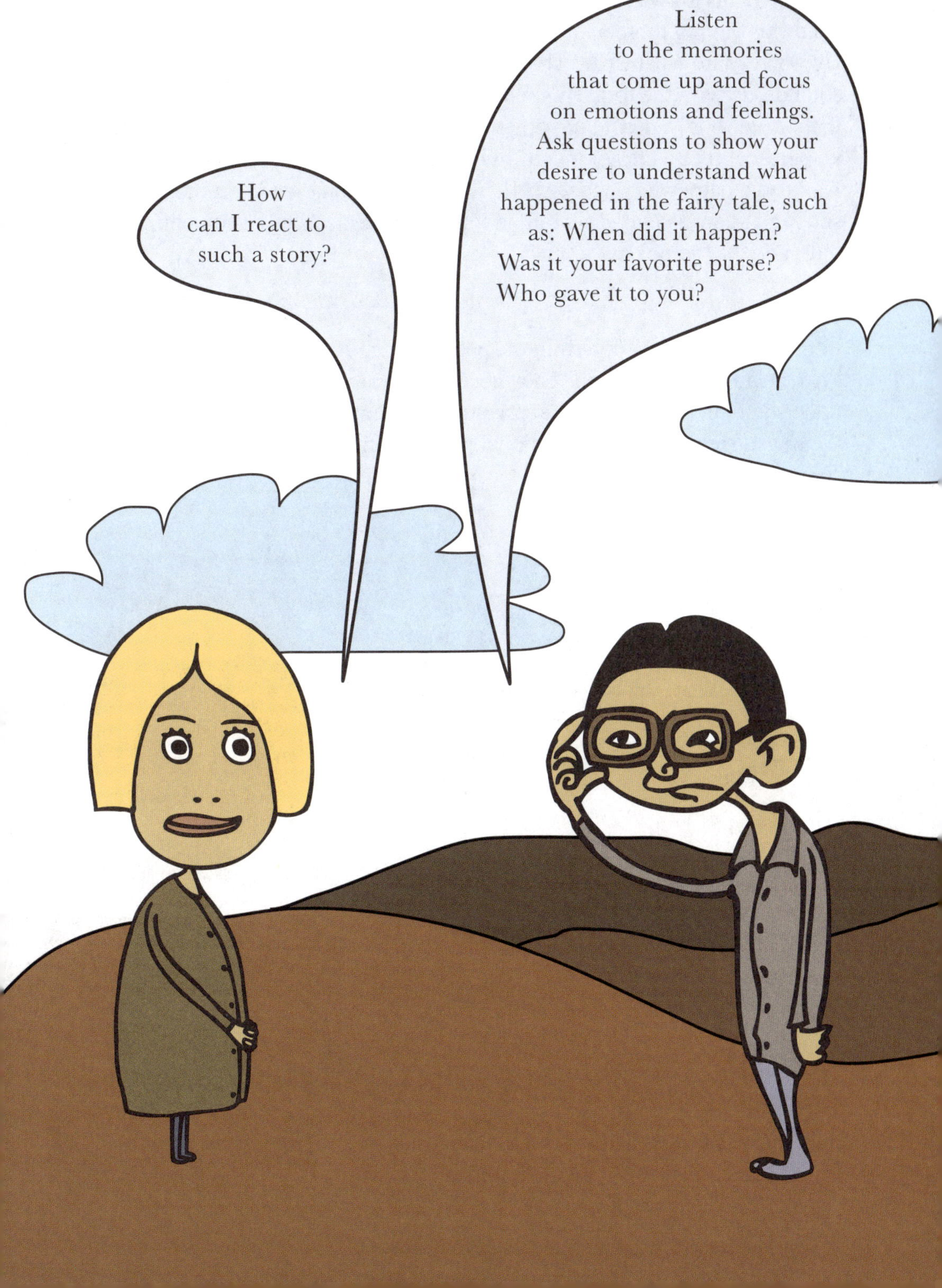
How can I react to such a story?
Listen to the memories that come up and focus on emotions and feelings. Ask questions to show your desire to understand what happened in the fairy tale, such as: When did it happen? Was it your favorite purse? Who gave it to you?

Where Is my Mom?

John was getting more and more anxious. He couldn't recognize this place. He wasn't sure what to do. Things around him looked unfamiliar. "What should I do with the fork? What do they want from me? I am hungry, but there is no food! I don't know these people. Where is my mom?!" Memories and present moments got mixed. John was here, now, a grown man, but he was also a baby who once was left alone for too long when his mom went shopping; he was five years old, in kindergarten, accused of something he didn't do: "Where is my mom?!"

Comment

In the later stages of forgetfulness, people often live inside their memories. Present and past are mixed. They need close emotional contact, love, and understanding. They need to express old feelings, and complete stories from their past. Help them find emotional peace. Remember: we all need a mom sometimes.

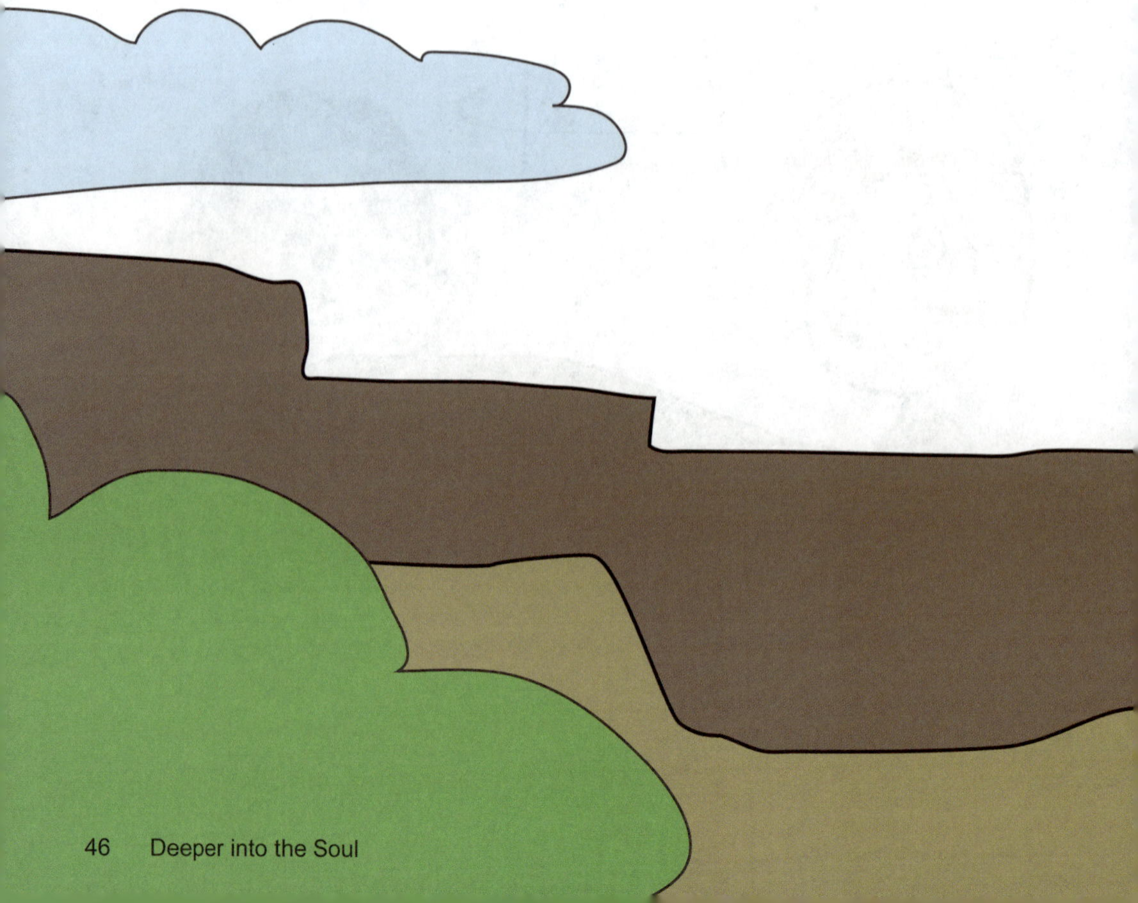

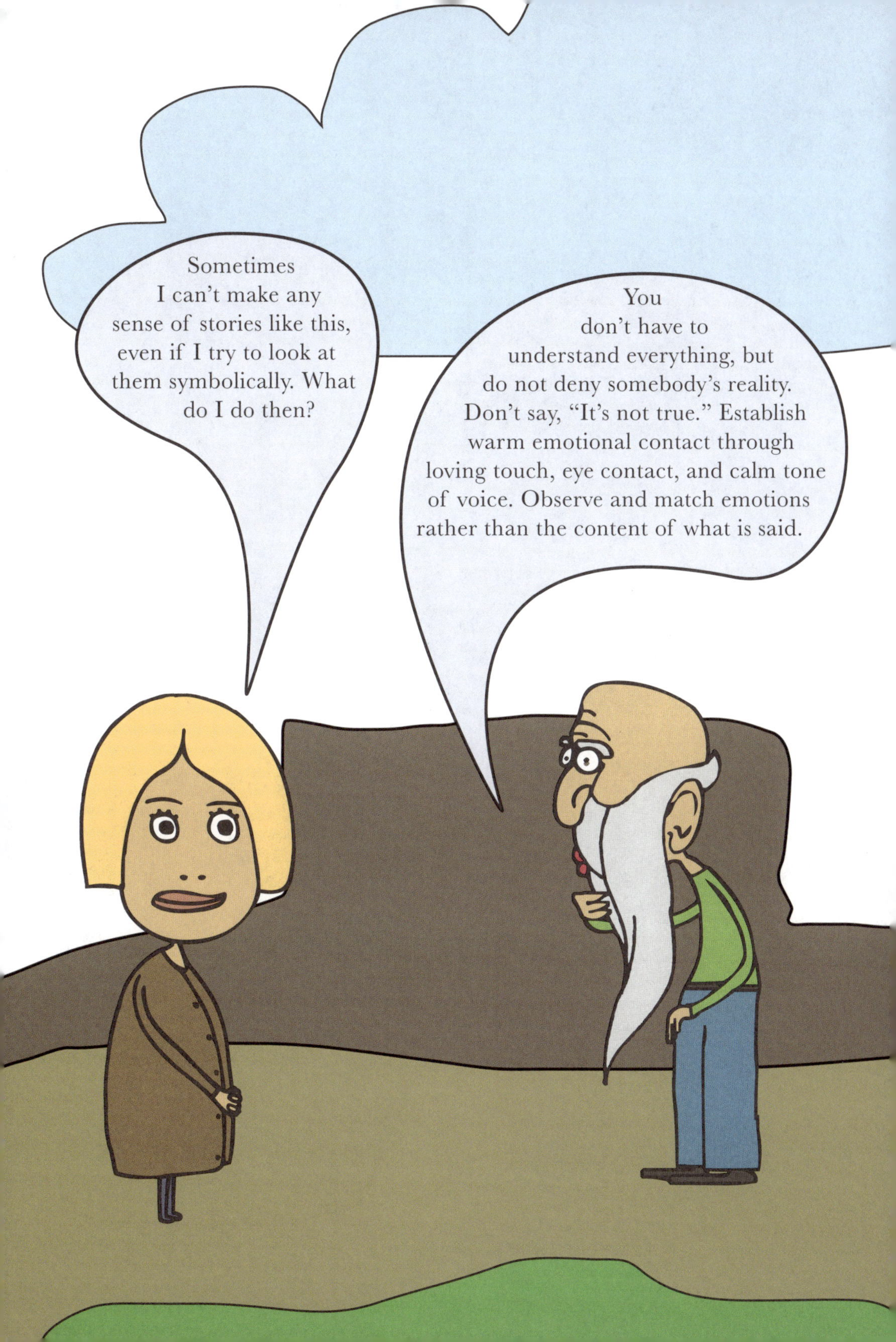
Sometimes I can't make any sense of stories like this, even if I try to look at them symbolically. What do I do then?
You don't have to understand everything, but do not deny somebody's reality. Don't say, "It's not true." Establish warm emotional contact through loving touch, eye contact, and calm tone of voice. Observe and match emotions rather than the content of what is said.

Part Two

Understanding Forgetfulness

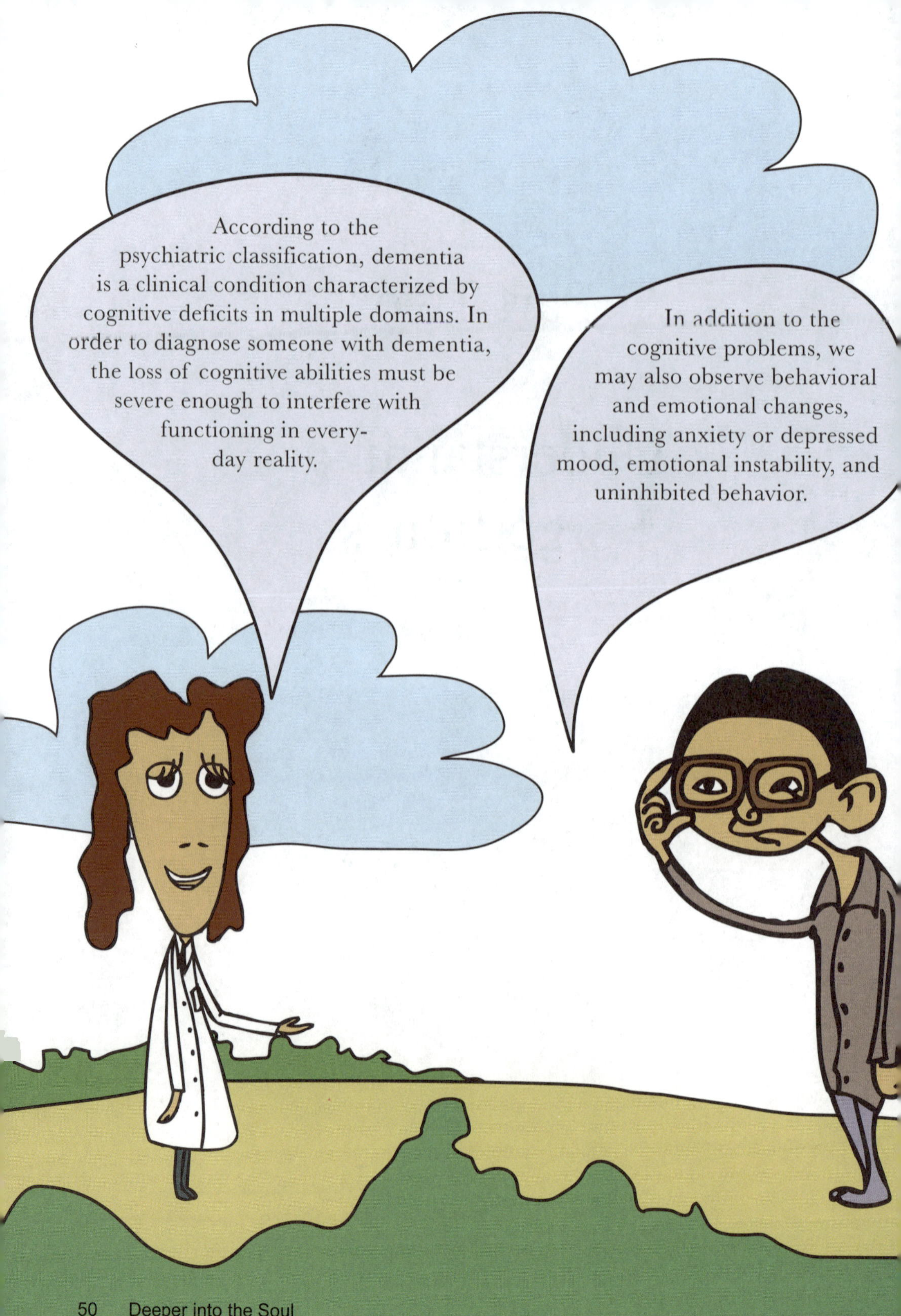
According to the psychiatric classification, dementia is a clinical condition characterized by cognitive deficits in multiple domains. In order to diagnose someone with dementia, the loss of cognitive abilities must be severe enough to interfere with functioning in every-day reality.
In addition to the cognitive problems, we may also observe behavioral and emotional changes, including anxiety or depressed mood, emotional instability, and uninhibited behavior.

Invitation

What we call forgetfulness has been described mostly in philosophical terms. In this section, we will look at the subject from the medical, biological perspective. At the same time, we hope to encourage a new attitude toward the world of forgetting.

We have to acknowledge the impressive achievements of contemporary science in gathering facts, creating and testing theories, formulating recommendations, and providing the means to alleviate some symptoms of dementia or at least slow its progress. In our book we present information in a broader context. Recent scientific research has helped us find the neurological foundation of various diseases associated with forgetfulness. Pharmacology continues to produce drugs that lessen the symptoms. Understanding the biological causes of certain behaviors that may seem bizarre from a commonsense point of view helps us to be less judgmental. We can see forgetfulness in the context of the individual as a biological organism affected by an illness.

With the help of our physician, Dr. Karen, we present the medical definition of dementia and some of its typical phases. We offer some basic information about the brain and the changes it undergoes during forgetfulness.

As we look at forgetfulness from a rational point of view, our Sage keeps reminding us of the mystery and of the unknown.

Medical Definitions

Dementia: What Does It Mean?

Let us look at the medical definitions of some terms that are commonly used in reference to people with forgetfulness. The term that labels the condition we call forgetfulness is dementia.

Forgetfulness (dementia)

- It is a progressive decline in mental functioning due to damage or disease in the brain.
- It is not a "disease" itself but a set of symptoms that may accompany different diseases.
- The changes in cognitive functioning are more profound than what is expected from normal aging.

Symptoms of forgetfulness (dementia)

The most prominent symptom is *memory impairment:*

- Difficulty learning new information.
- Forgetting what has been recently learned.

Forgetfulness typically includes at least one of the following:

- Aphasia
    - Difficulty finding and using words.
    - Difficulty understanding language.

- Agnosia
    - Difficulty recognizing and identifying objects.

- Apraxia
    - Loss of ability to carry out skilled movement or gestures.
    - Disturbance in planning, reasoning, and controlling behavior.
    - Difficulty in understanding and following direction.

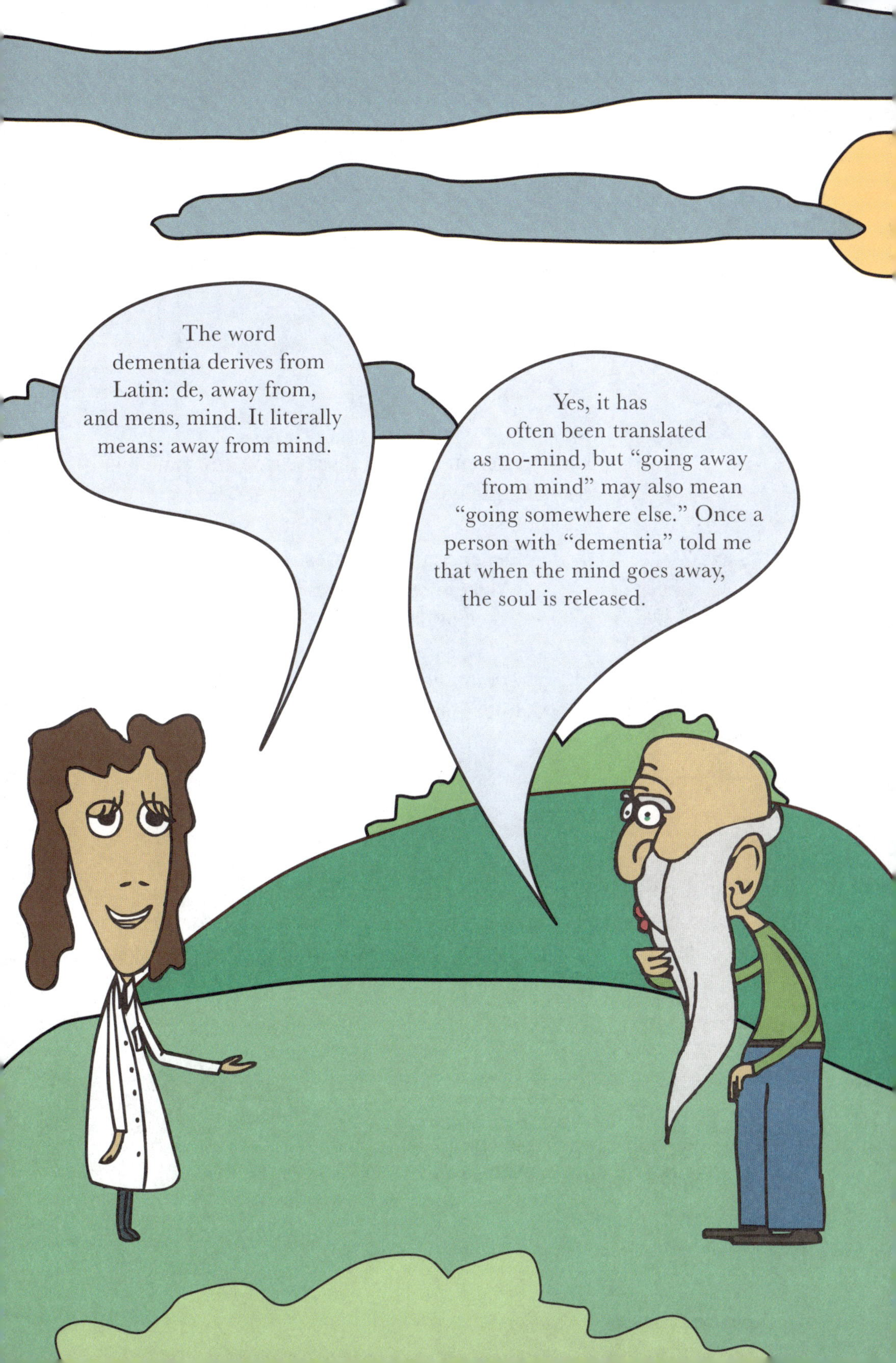
The word dementia derives from Latin: de, away from, and mens, mind. It literally means: away from mind.
Yes, it has often been translated as no-mind, but “going away from mind” may also mean “going somewhere else.” Once a person with “dementia” told me that when the mind goes away, the soul is released.

Types of Forgetfulness

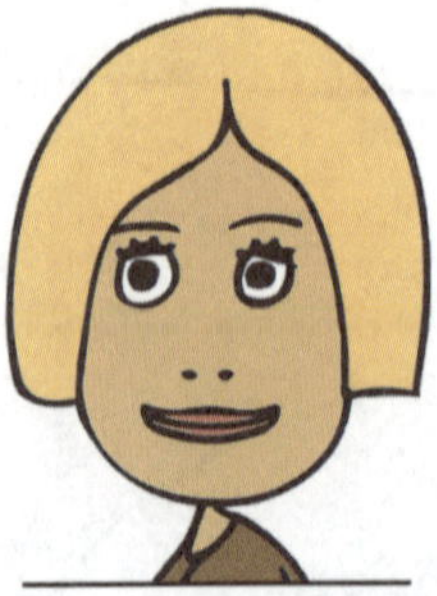

What are the causes of forgetfulness from the medical point of view?

Many different types of diseases are associated with forgetfulness, including:

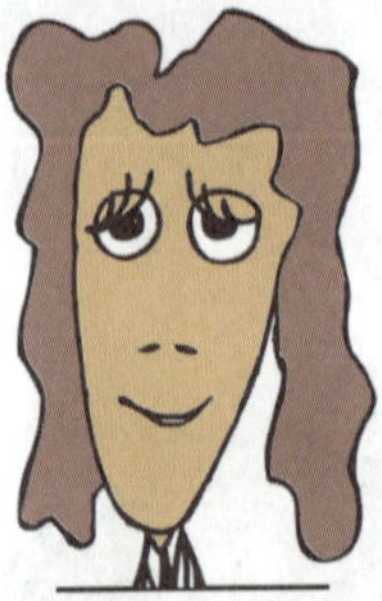

- Degenerative diseases (Alzheimer's disease, Pick's disease).
- Vascular dementia (multi-infarct dementia).
- Traumatic dementia (Boxer's dementia).
- Infectious dementia (Creutzfeldt-Jakob disease).
- Toxic dementia (alcoholic dementia).

It is estimated that Alzheimer's disease, also called dementia of Alzheimer's type, is the most common cause of forgetfulness, accounting for 50 to 75 percent of all dementia cases. Vascular dementia is the second most common. Let's look at the two of them.

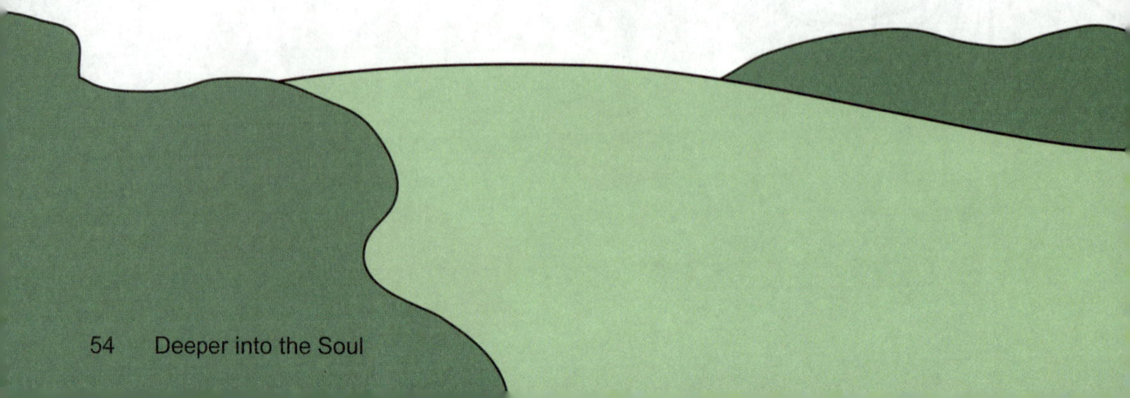

Alzheimer's Disease

- *What happens in the brain?*
  Brain cells (neurons) and spaces between them become clogged with protein deposits, called plaques and tangles. These plaques and tangles prevent neurons from sending information to each other. Eventually, neurons in different parts of the brain die.

- *How does it affect cognitive functioning?*
  The first part of the brain affected is the hippocampus, the section responsible for short-term memory. Thus the first symptom is forgetting recent information. People with Alzheimer's disease progressively lose the ability to remember new material, to recognize people, places, and objects, to find and understand words, and to carry out simple activities such as eating or dressing.

- *When does it start?*
  Alzheimer's disease typically begins after age 60.

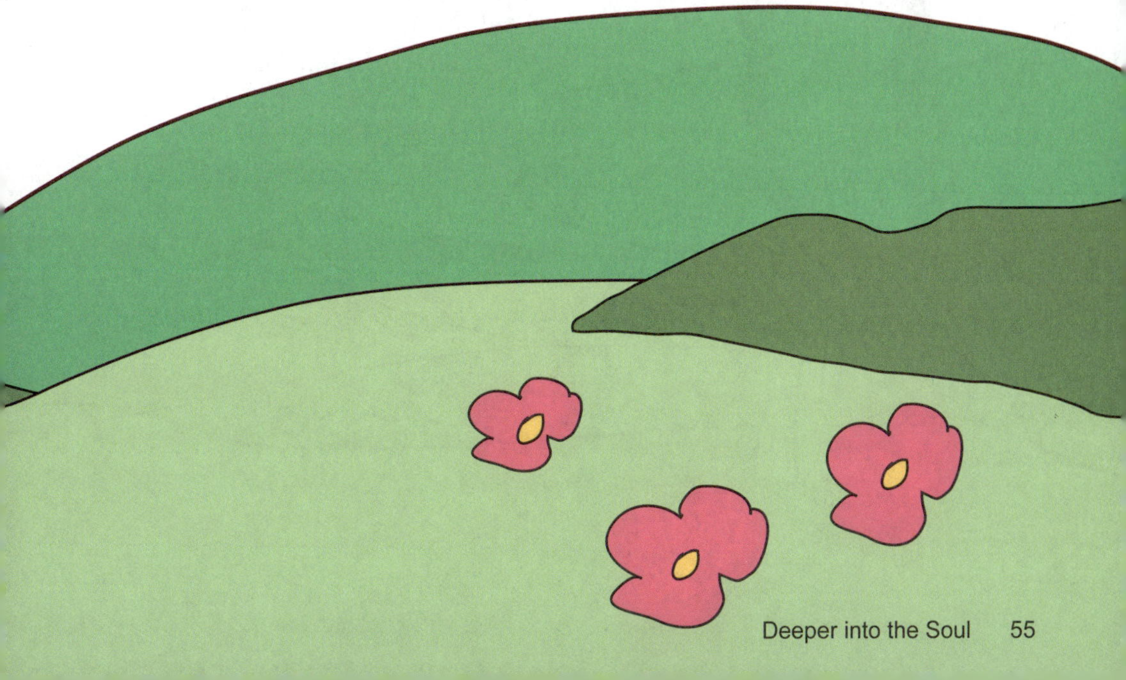

Vascular Dementia

- *What happens in the brain?*
  The vessels in the brain become blocked by blood clots or fatty deposits; blood cannot get to parts of the brain and a stroke occurs. A stroke can also occur when the vessel bursts. A series of strokes disrupts blood flow and damages or destroys brain tissue.

- *How does it affect cognitive functioning?*
  Patterns of cognitive decline in vascular dementia are difficult to predict. Depending on which parts of the brain have been destroyed, some functions may be impaired while others may be relatively unaffected for a while.

- *When does it start?*
  Vascular dementia may begin any time later in life, though it is less common after 75.

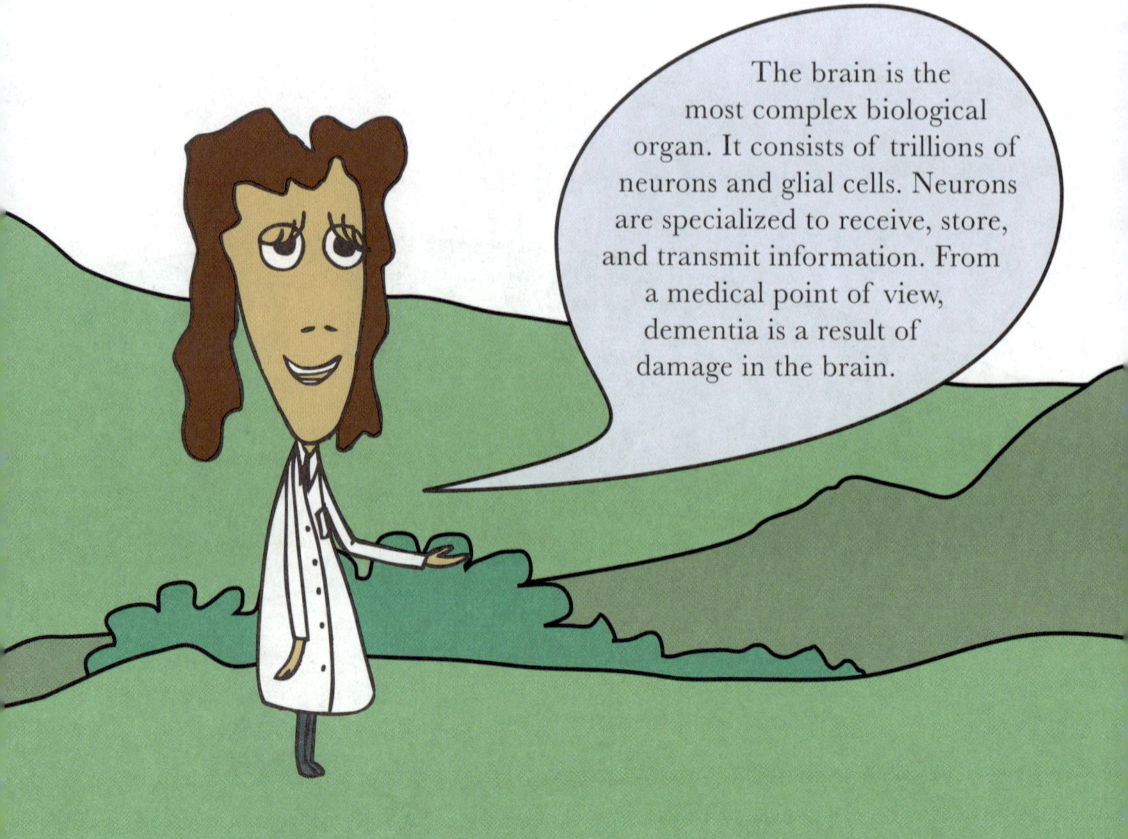
The brain is the most complex biological organ. It consists of trillions of neurons and glial cells. Neurons are specialized to receive, store, and transmit information. From a medical point of view, dementia is a result of damage in the brain.

Emotions Remain: Brain Changes in Forgetfulness

As we are trying to understand the brain by using the brain itself, we are a long way from a clear definition of the mind and consciousness. How do impulses become thoughts? How is memory stored? What is the connection between mental activities and feelings?

—Comment at the scientific international exhibition "Brain"

Different areas of the brain are responsible for different skills or abilities (though sometimes other areas may take over when one part is damaged). As expected, then, the changes we see in people with Alzheimer's type dementia are related to the parts of the brain that have been affected. Let's look at some basic functions of different parts of the brain. We offer examples of common problems associated with these specific parts of the brain, as well as the sorts of difficulties a person with Alzheimer's may face.

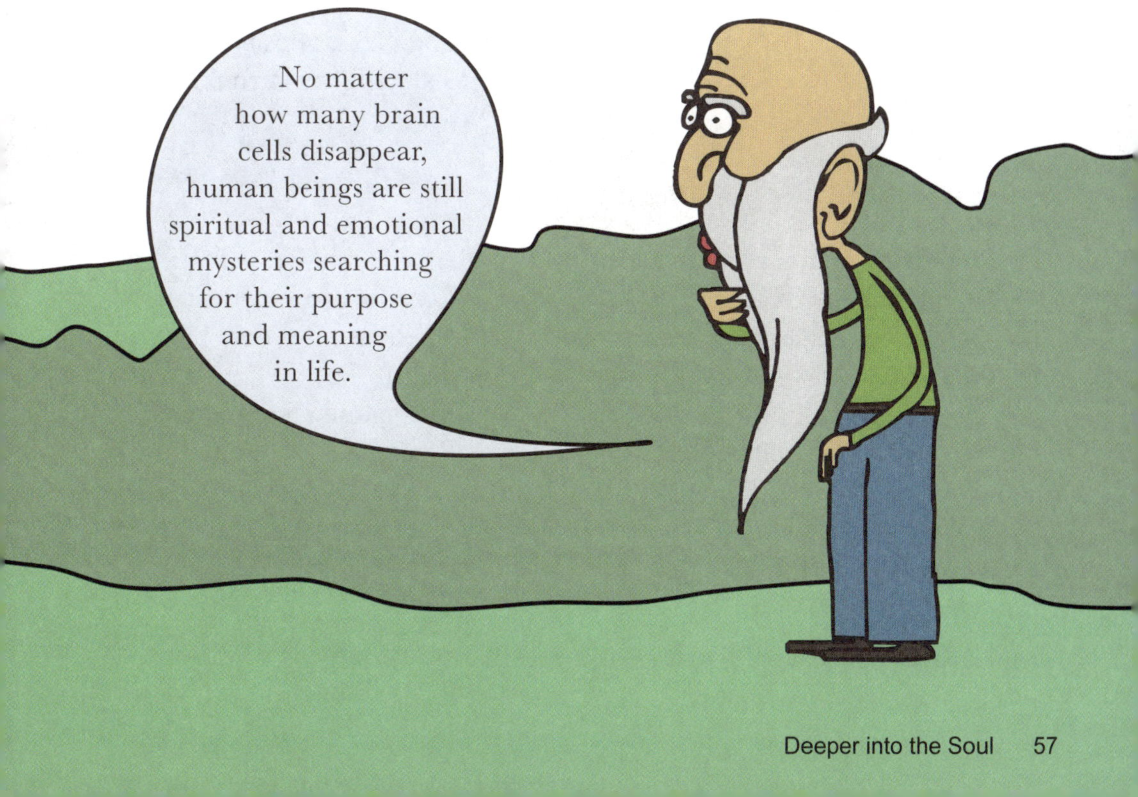

Hippocampus
- Short-term memory.
- New learning.

Everyone: forgetting your ATM pin number.
Alzheimer's: forgetting the purpose of your ATM card.

Temporal Lobe
- Understanding spoken words.
- Finding appropriate words.
- Hearing ability.

Everyone: not able to think of a specific, descriptive word.
Alzheimer's: not able to remember simple nouns such as "cup".

Occipital Lobe
- Visual perception and interpretation of visual clues.
- Depth perception.
- Recognition of faces and objects.

Everyone: not recognizing a face of a well-known actress in a magazine.
Alzheimer's: not recognizing the face of your own daughter in a family photo.

Frontal Lobe
- Judgment.
- Reasoning and decision making.
- Looking inward, understanding oneself and others.
- Controlling and planning actions and emotions.

Everyone: saying you don't like a food you haven't tried.
Alzheimer's: refusing to eat food while insisting it has been poisoned.

Parietal Lobe
- Processing spatial relationships.
- Orienting body in space.
- Finding out what and where things are.

Everyone: taking one book for another.
Alzheimer's: insisting on using a television for a computer.

Amygdala
(remains relatively unaffected)
- Evoking and experiencing emotions (not controlling them).
- Responding to emotions.
- Perceiving emotions.

Inspired by http://www.pbs.org/theforgetting/symptoms/index.html

Even those with Alzheimer's disease can achieve higher emotional levels (feelings of belonging, positive mood, and contact with their real Self). One of the last parts of the brain affected by the disease, the amygdala, receives, reacts to, and expresses mood and emotion. Mood and emotion are therefore readily accessible to caregivers until very late in the disease.

– Paul Raia, *Habilitation Therapy*

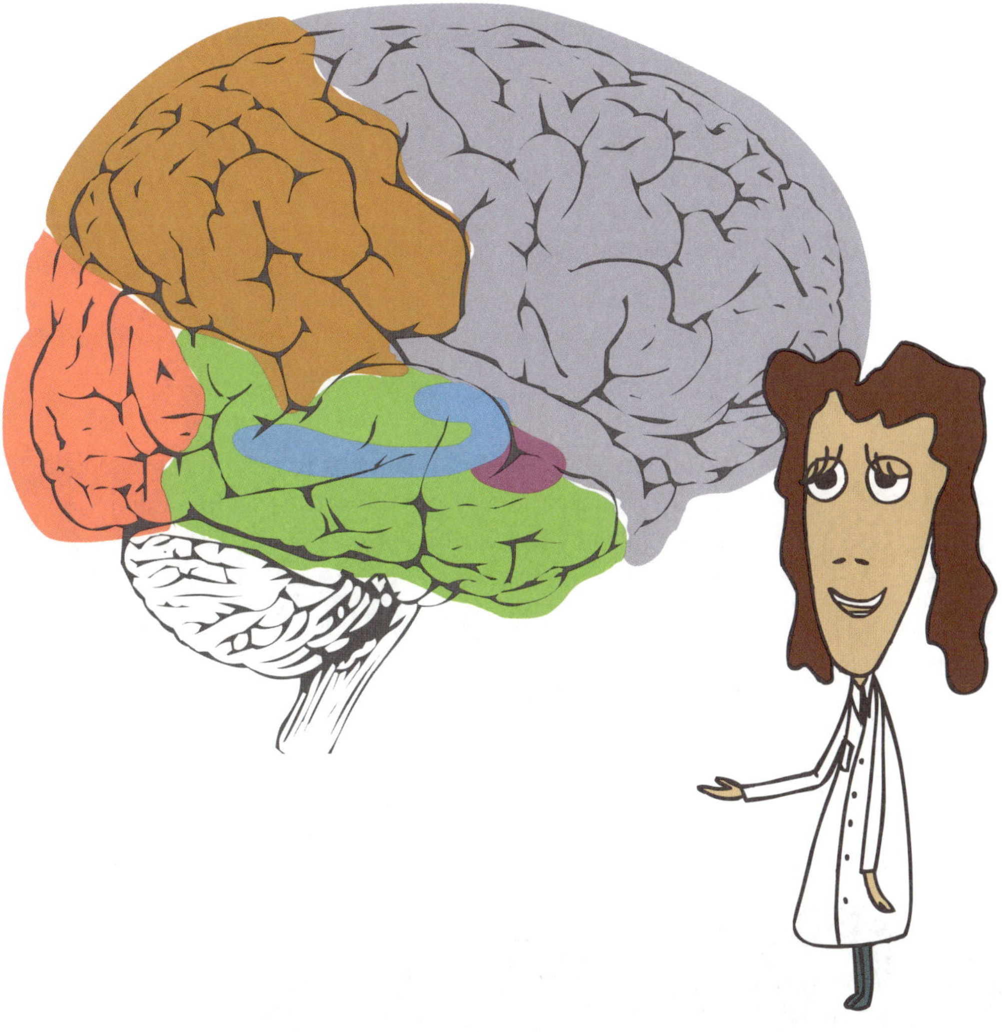

Different Phases, Different Needs

People with forgetfulness change over time. There are, of course, individual differences in the patterns of these changes. Some functions may become worse and then better again within a short period, sometimes within one day. However, forgetfulness is a progressive condition, and certain changes can be expected over time.

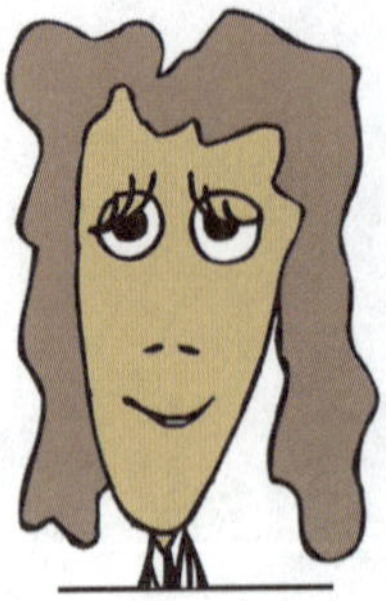

Features of dementia are commonly classified into three stages:

- Mild.
- Moderate.
- Severe.

Note: Sometimes a fourth stage, "profound dementia," is added.

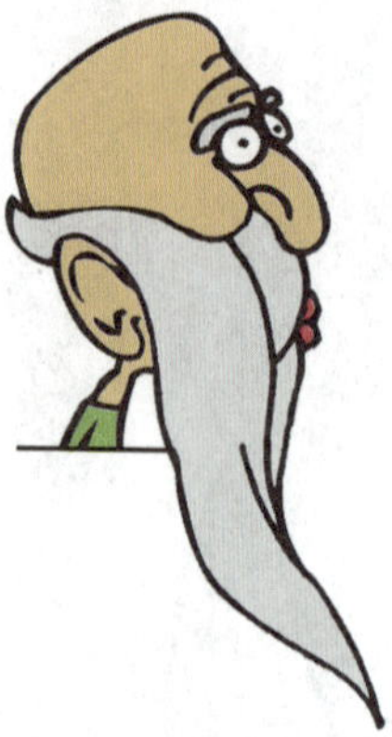

We understand different phases of forgetfulness as being closer or further away from consensus reality. Each human journey has various phases. Each part of the journey is as important and meaningful as any other. It is up to us to see this. Being in our "everyday reality" is not any more important than being in Dreamland or getting in touch with the Essence.

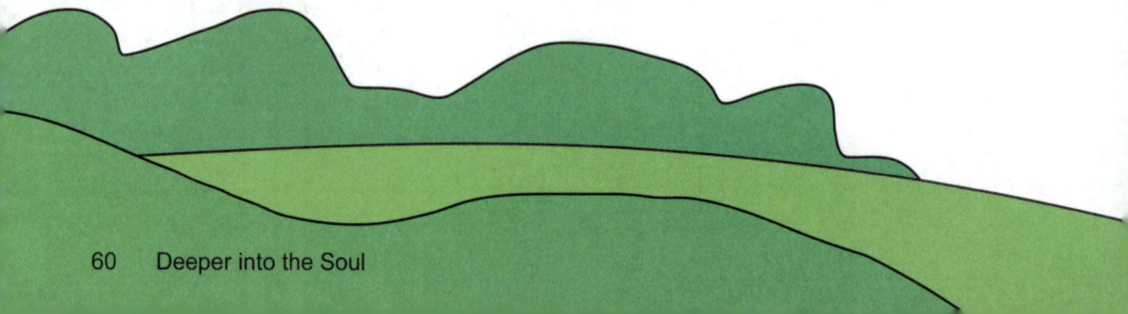

Phases of Forgetfulness

I. *Departure from Consensus Reality*

People in the early stages of Alzheimer's (mild dementia):

- Notice their short-term memory does not function as before.
- Feel bad about getting lost or confused.
- Get worried.
- Try to stay close to everyday reality and get anxious when things become difficult.
- Judge themselves according to our social and intellectual standards.
- Have trouble remembering recent events.
- Have difficulty learning new information about everyday reality.
- Forget names.
- Lose concentration.
- Have a tendency to lose things.
- Lose orientation in time (date, month, year).
- Withdraw from social contact.
- Have difficulty planning or making judgments or decisions in consensus reality.

Recommendations for caregivers:
- Do not confront a person with his memory and learning problems.
- Do acknowledge what she can do in everyday reality.

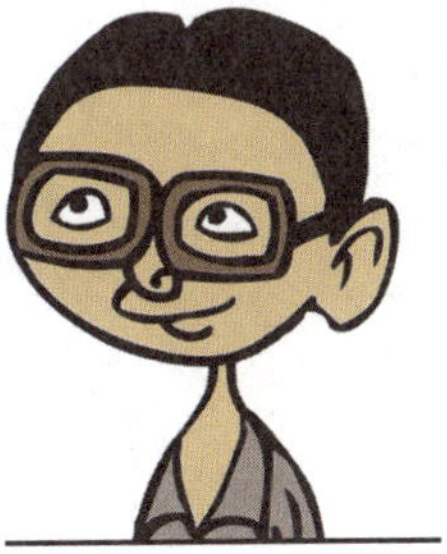

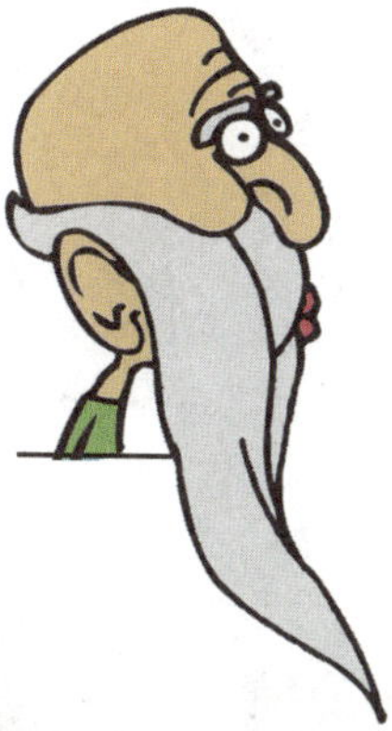

- Old people often use an object like a wedding ring to symbolize something from the past.
- A person in present time, like yourself, can represent a mother or sister.
- When old people combine one thought with another they are often very poetic.

II. ***Between the Worlds***

People in the middle stage of Alzheimer's (moderate dementia) tend to:

- Live more and more in their dream-like worlds.
- Confuse past and present.
- Begin to lose their command of what is appropriate and what is not.
- See themselves as "oriented in an unknown world" rather than "disoriented in a known world."
- Have increasing difficulty using spoken language.
- Display strong emotions, such as fear and anger.
- Communicate through repeated movements.
- Pace and wander.
- Exhibit behaviors we don't understand and don't know how to respond to.
- Lose some ability to read and write.
- Lose coordination.
- Have difficulty with spatial orientation.
- Have difficulty with everyday activities, such as eating, dressing, and bathing.
- Experience incontinence.

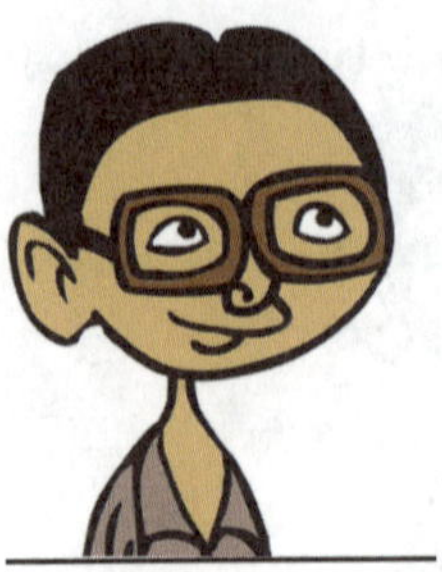

Recommendations for caregivers:

- Try to create a calm, relaxed atmosphere.
- Avoid too much stimulation.
- Expect sudden outbursts of emotions: observe early signs, understand and explore what they mean.
- Allow as much independence as possible while creating a structure that minimizes confusion.
- Do not reason or argue.
- Be curious about each emotion and each type of behavior: look at it as a creative expression of human spirit and try to understand its symbolic meaning.

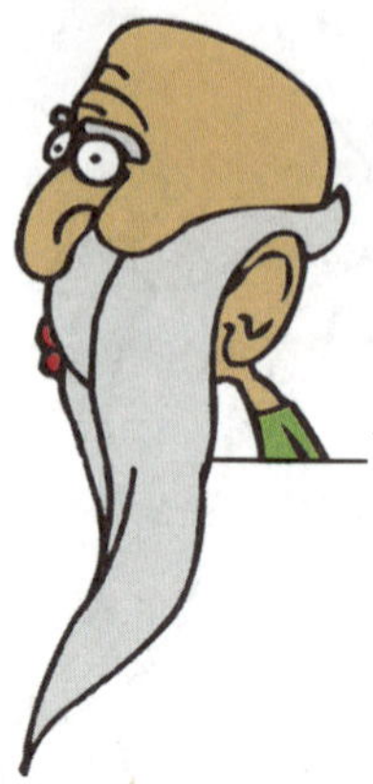

III. ***In the Other Reality***

People in the late stage of Alzheimer's (severe dementia) tend to:

- Not recognize places, people, or objects in consensus reality.
- Not communicate verbally with us.
- Have muscles that are often tense.
- Be unable to walk.
- Need a lot of help with personal care.
- Spend most of their time in Dreamland (sleeping, daydreaming, attention inward).
- Have incontinence.
- Experience weight loss.

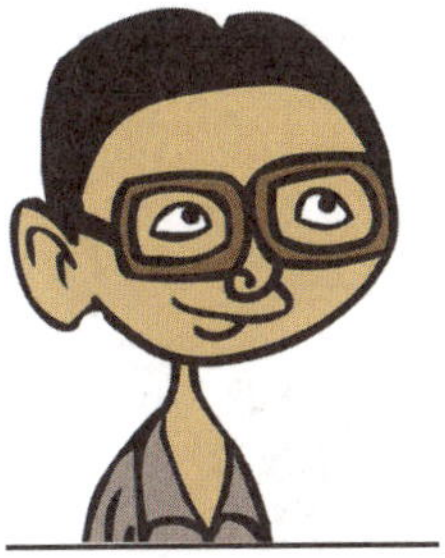

Recommendations for caregivers:

- Respect the dignity of the body.
- Never talk about a person as if she is not present.
- Be gentle.

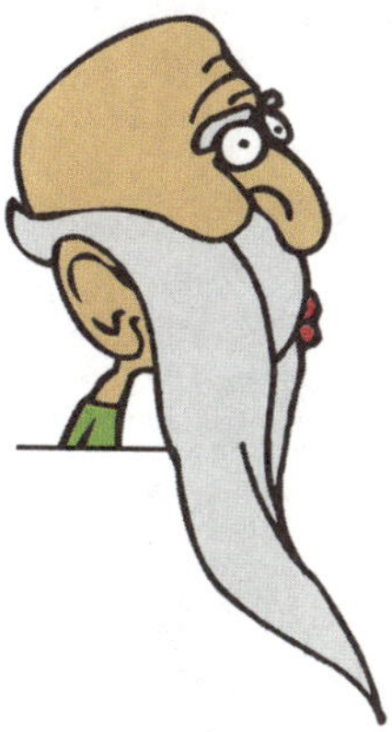

- Remember that a person is spiritually and emotionally present: we are all spiritual beings at each moment of our lives.

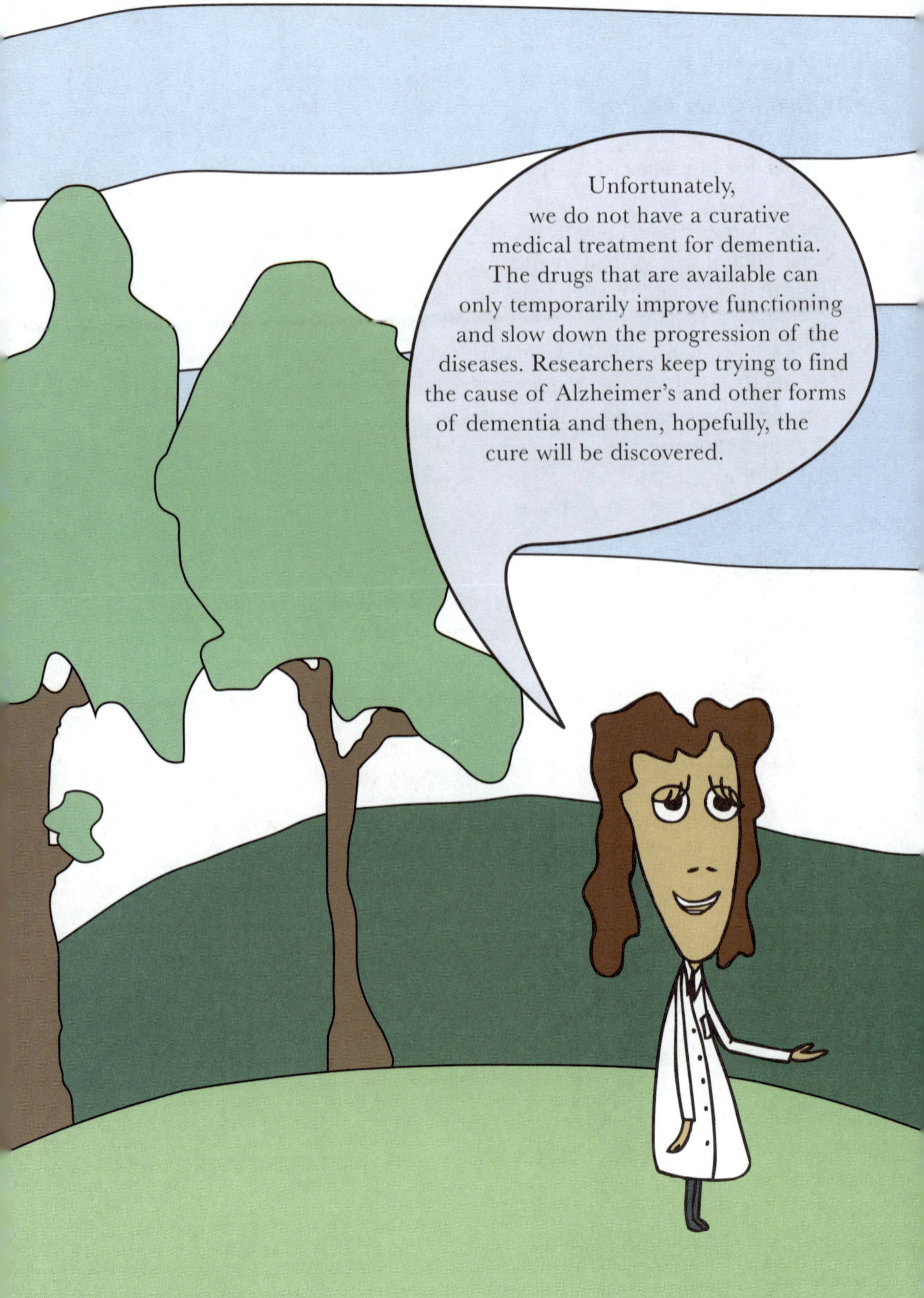
Unfortunately, we do not have a curative medical treatment for dementia. The drugs that are available can only temporarily improve functioning and slow down the progression of the diseases. Researchers keep trying to find the cause of Alzheimer's and other forms of dementia and then, hopefully, the cure will be discovered.

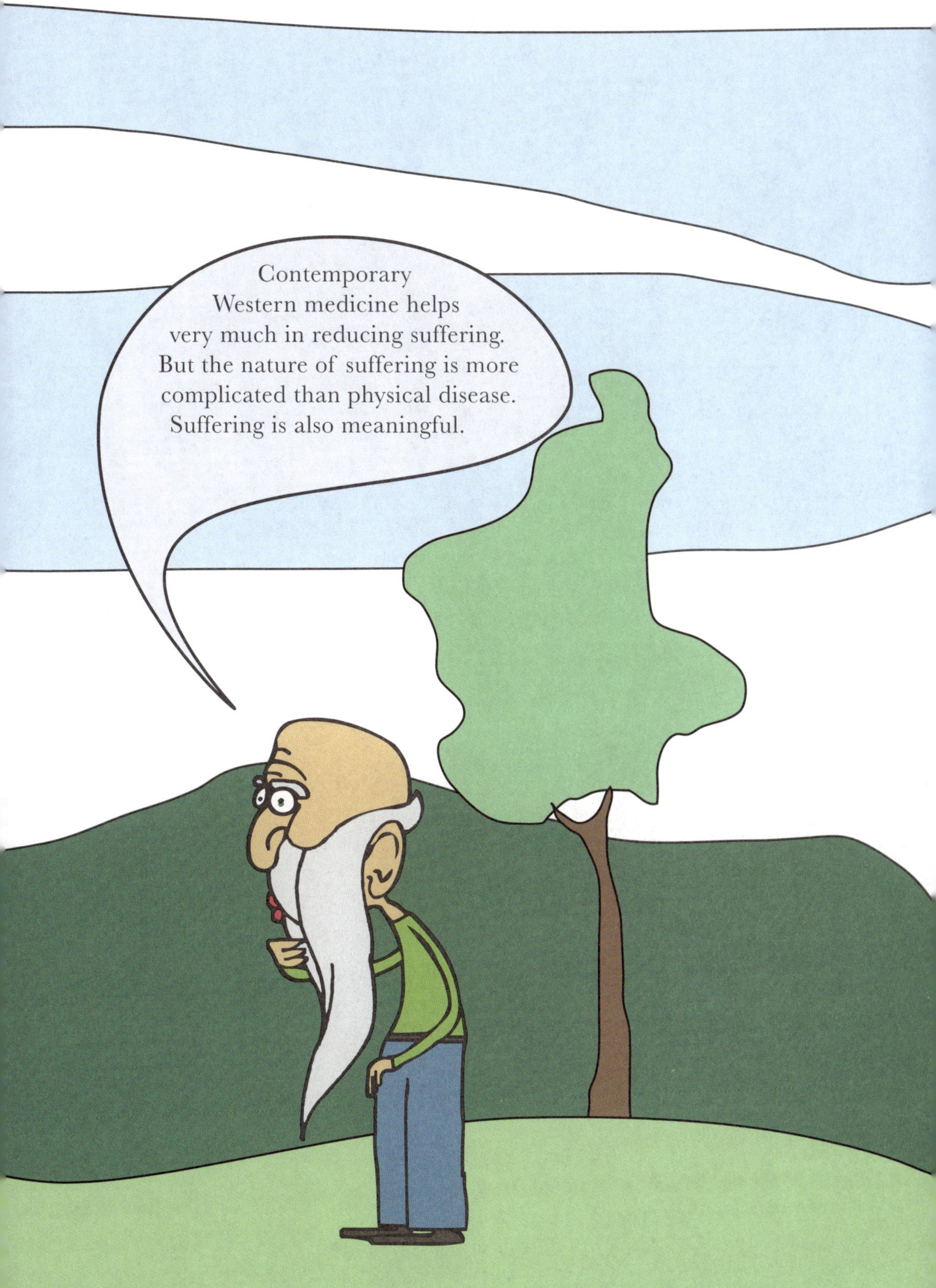
Contemporary Western medicine helps very much in reducing suffering. But the nature of suffering is more complicated than physical disease. Suffering is also meaningful.

Part Three

Learning Skills

Invitation

Being with and caring for a person with Forgetfulness confronts us with the unexpected and unknown. Many publications have asserted that people with Alzheimer's disease suffer a "tragic loss of a person" and undergo "dramatic changes in personality."

People with Dementia are often called "victims" of a disease. As a leading figure in Dementia care, Naomi Feil, told us: "I find that these people are not victims. They are often wiser than those who call them victims."

Here, we try to see changes due to forgetting and disorientation not as tragic but as yet another chance to enter more deeply into our soul for both the caregiver and the person with symptoms of forgetfulness. We look not only at what is lost, but also at what is gained.

We encourage openness toward this new, emerging person, even if his or her behavior seems "weird." We recommend that caregivers stay open to the world of forgetting and to their own feelings and questions. In Part Two, we offered some medical information about forgetfulness to help our rational minds better understand the person who keeps changing. But we must go beyond what's called reason. Openness, love, curiosity and acceptance seem to be key attitudes.

Yet, these attitudes are difficult to maintain. Days are filled with quarrels or full-blown outbursts of unexpected emotions. The people we care for disappear into their "world of forgetting," sometimes literally leave the house and wander off.

In addition to an open attitude and some rational knowledge, we need communication skills. In this section we present some suggestions to make daily life easier. We discuss how to communicate with a person with forgetfulness. We also address communication among caregivers.

Remember: we are learning together here. We are only just beginning to understand the many experiences of forgetfulness, of our journey into the soul.

Communicating with a Person with Forgetfulness Symptoms

Being Together in the Flow of Signals

Everything we do in our interactions with other people is a part of communication flow. Our words, facial expressions, tone of voice, and body language all carry a message. As Bateson, Watzlawick and others point out, some messages we send consciously, usually the content of what we communicate. When we say, "The tea is ready," we also send much other information through tone of voice, facial expression, distance, posture, and gestures. With such "relationship messages," we reveal our feelings toward the other person. We may say, "The tea is ready" angrily or warmly; we may turn our back or gently hold the person's hand. Remember, people who are less present in our consensus reality are often much more sensitive to relationship messages. They are focused less on content than on feelings.

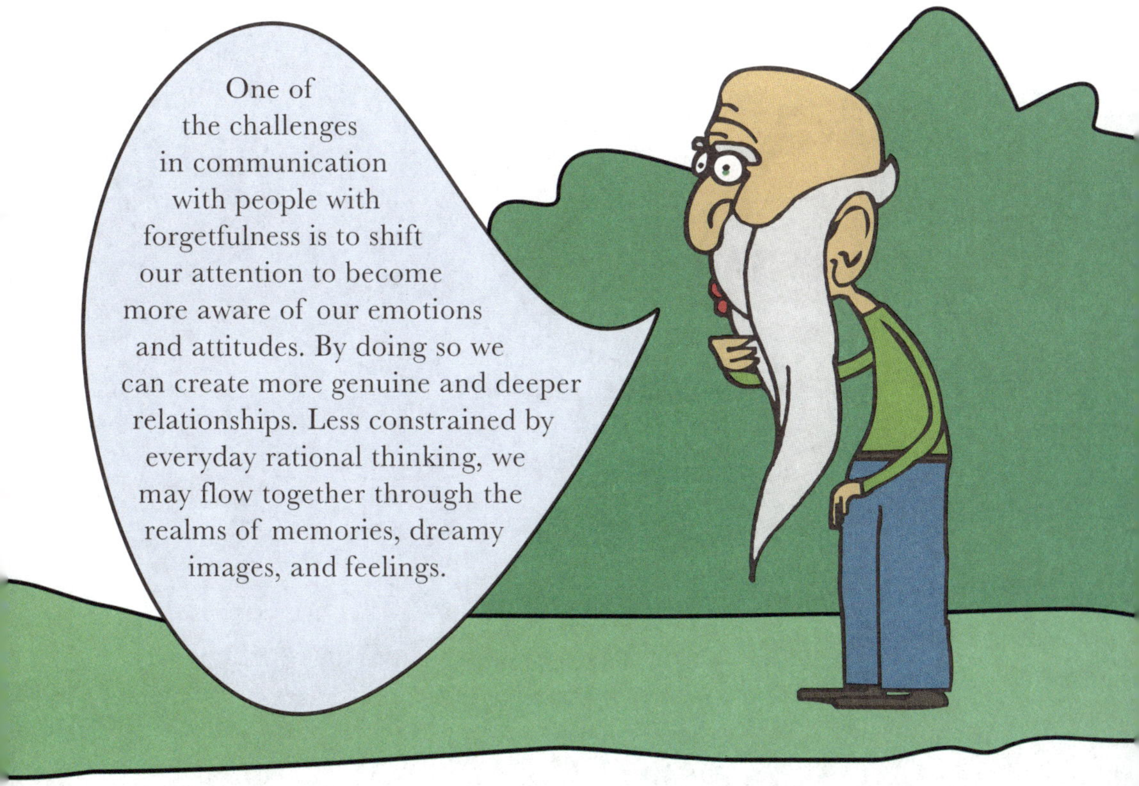

First Moments Create the Atmosphere

Before You Start

- Get centered (take a few deep breaths, meditate for a few minutes).
- Create a warm positive mood (notice the beauty of the person, think about his good intentions).
- Minimize distractions (such as loud music, TV, or nearby conversation).
- Don't pretend to be nice when you are angry; take a moment to calm down and relax.
- Try to see the situation through the eyes of the person with symptoms of forgetfulness.
- Practice empathy and acceptance.
- Focus on emotions and feelings.
- Show affection and reassurance.

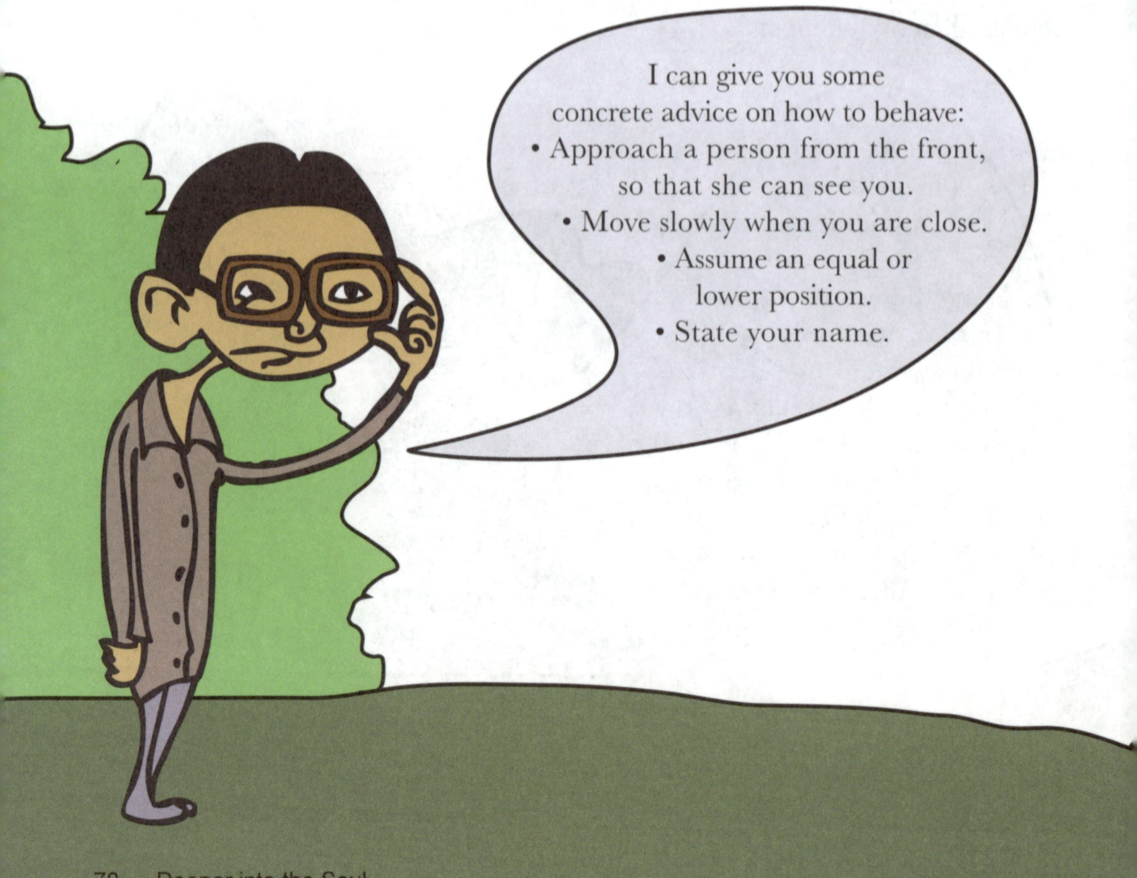
I can give you some concrete advice on how to behave:
• Approach a person from the front, so that she can see you.
• Move slowly when you are close.
• Assume an equal or lower position.
• State your name.

Nonverbal Communication

- Try to convey the message with your words, your tone, and your facial expression.
- Avoid sudden movements.
- Give visual cues or write things down.
- Use a soft, calm voice.
- Speak slowly.
- Listen with your ears, eyes, heart, and soul.
- Show your affection and reassurance.

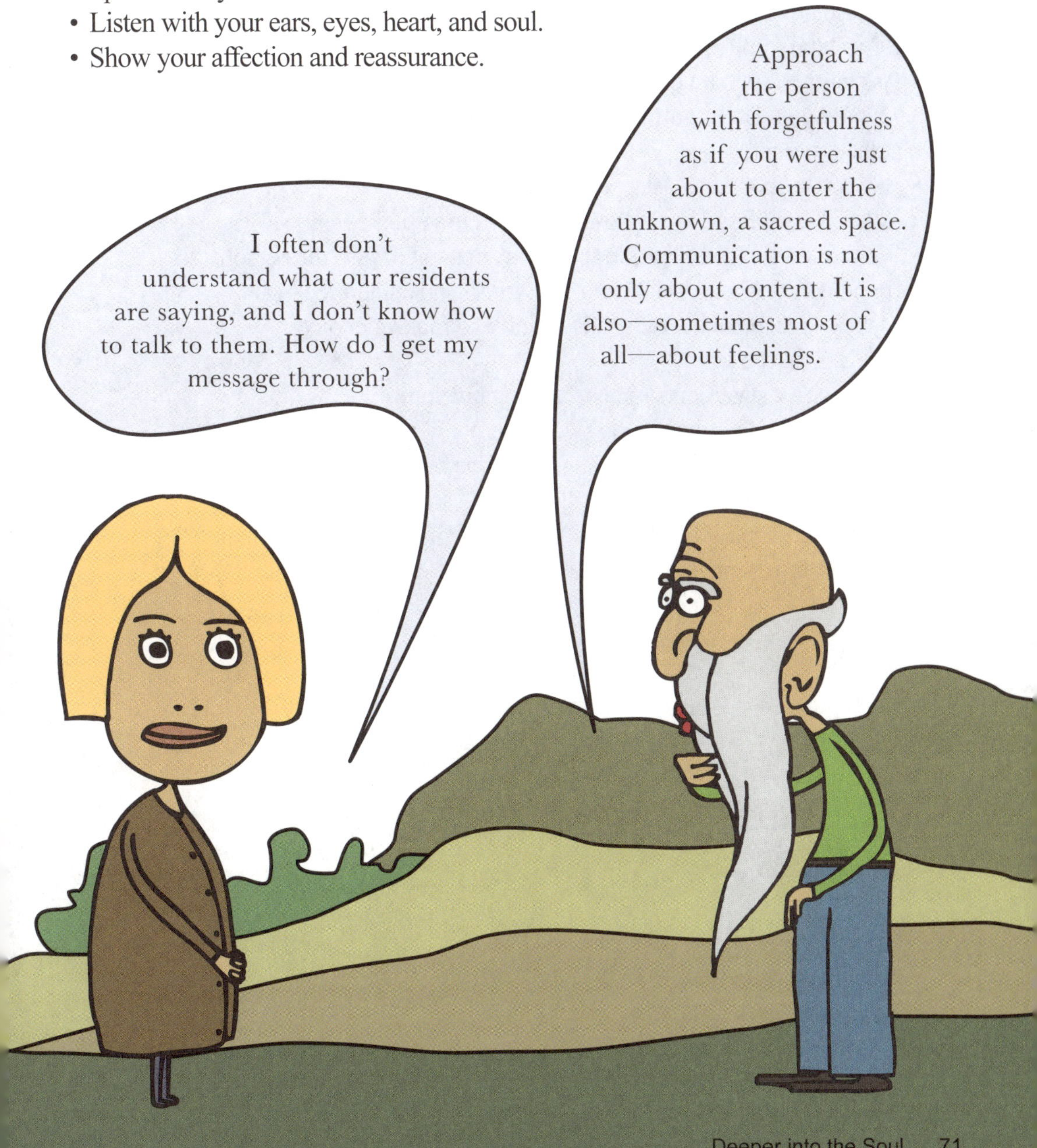
I often don't understand what our residents are saying, and I don't know how to talk to them. How do I get my message through?
Approach the person with forgetfulness as if you were just about to enter the unknown, a sacred space. Communication is not only about content. It is also—sometimes most of all—about feelings.

Verbal Communication

Yes

- Use simple statements:
  "Here is your tea," rather than "I have prepared a cup of tea for you, but I wasn't sure if you wanted herb tea or black tea."
- Use concrete phrases:
  "Please put your T-shirt on," rather than "Get dressed."
- Repeat the same phrase if needed.
- Ask simple, specific questions:
  "Would you like to go for a walk?" rather than "What do you feel like doing at the moment?"
- As you walk outside, ask specific questions:
  "Would you like to see yellow flowers? Do you like yellow?"
- Wait for an answer; do not press if it seems to confuse the person.
- If you don't understand the content, try to understand feelings.
- Make suggestions if a person is not able to make a choice:
  "Let's go to the patio."
- Use positive statements rather than negative ones:
  "Stay here" rather than "Don't go there."
- If it gets difficult, stop and try another time.
- Limit choices to minimize confusion:
  "Here is an apple," rather than "What kind of a fruit would you like?"
- Use humor whenever possible.

No

- Do not give more than one instruction at a time:
  "Please put on your socks now," rather than "First put on your T-shirt, then your sweater, and when you are done with that, let's go have some tea."
- Do not argue or reason.
- Avoid lengthy verbal instructions.
- Don't use complex sentences or vocabulary.
- Don't try to persuade the person that he is wrong:
  don't say, "Nobody has stolen your glasses; you must have put them somewhere and now you don't remember."
- Don't make judgmental comments about the person's forgetting, such as, "It's really annoying that you can't remember where you left your book!"
- Don't criticize or reproach: "You shouldn't take off your pants in the corridor; a gentleman like you shouldn't be doing such things in public!"

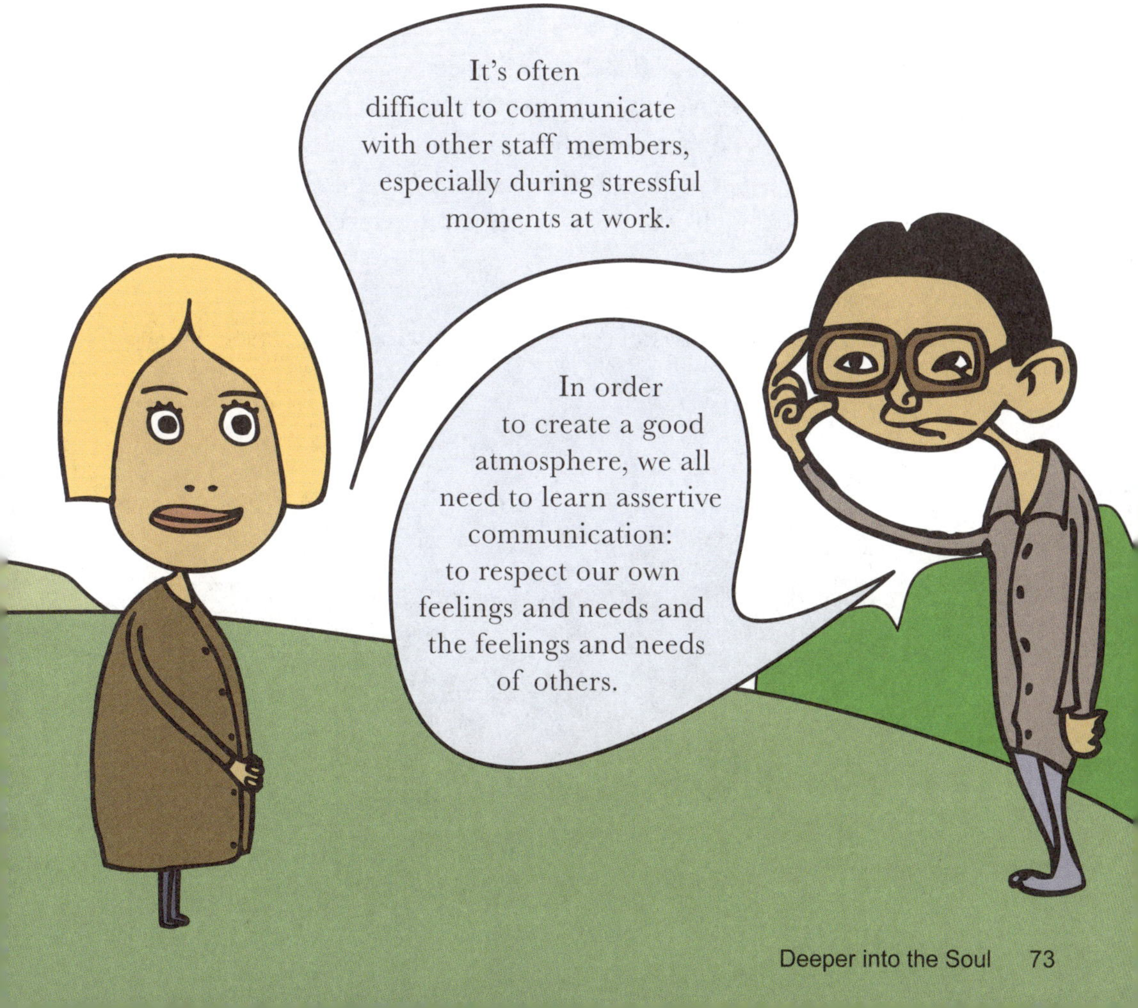
It's often difficult to communicate with other staff members, especially during stressful moments at work.
In order to create a good atmosphere, we all need to learn assertive communication: to respect our own feelings and needs and the feelings and needs of others.

Teamwork

If you work in a residential facility, the team you are part of may be both a source of support and a source of frustration. To get the most out of teamwork, we first need to learn to communicate with each other.

Learn to Express Yourself

- Learn to express your needs and feelings using "I messages"—say "I am angry" rather than "you make me angry."
- Do not assume that the other person will guess what you need.
- Be clear and direct—take a risk: if you express your need directly, the other may say "yes" or "no" to it, but you will understand one another better.
- Learn to say "no"—listen to your instincts.
- If you are not sure about your immediate response, say, "I need to think about it first."

Learn to Listen to Others

- Learn to listen to the needs and feelings of others.
- Focus on what other people are trying to express.
- Always look for the good intentions behind words.
- Differentiate between immediate behavior and the character of a person—say "I do not like it when you raise your voice" rather than "You are such a harsh person."
- Allow others to express their feelings.
- Respect personal space—do not come too close or disturb a person who needs a moment of privacy.

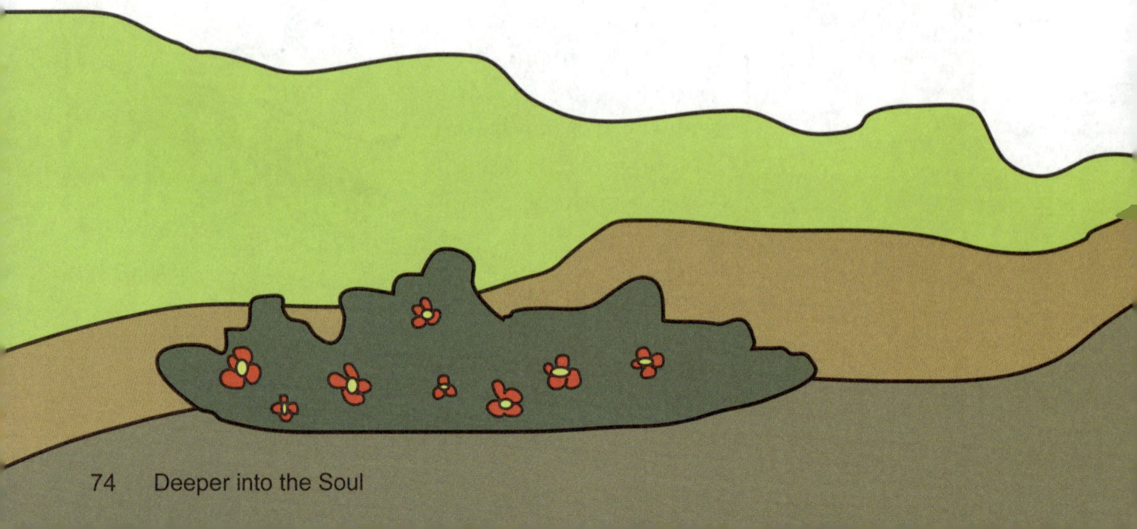

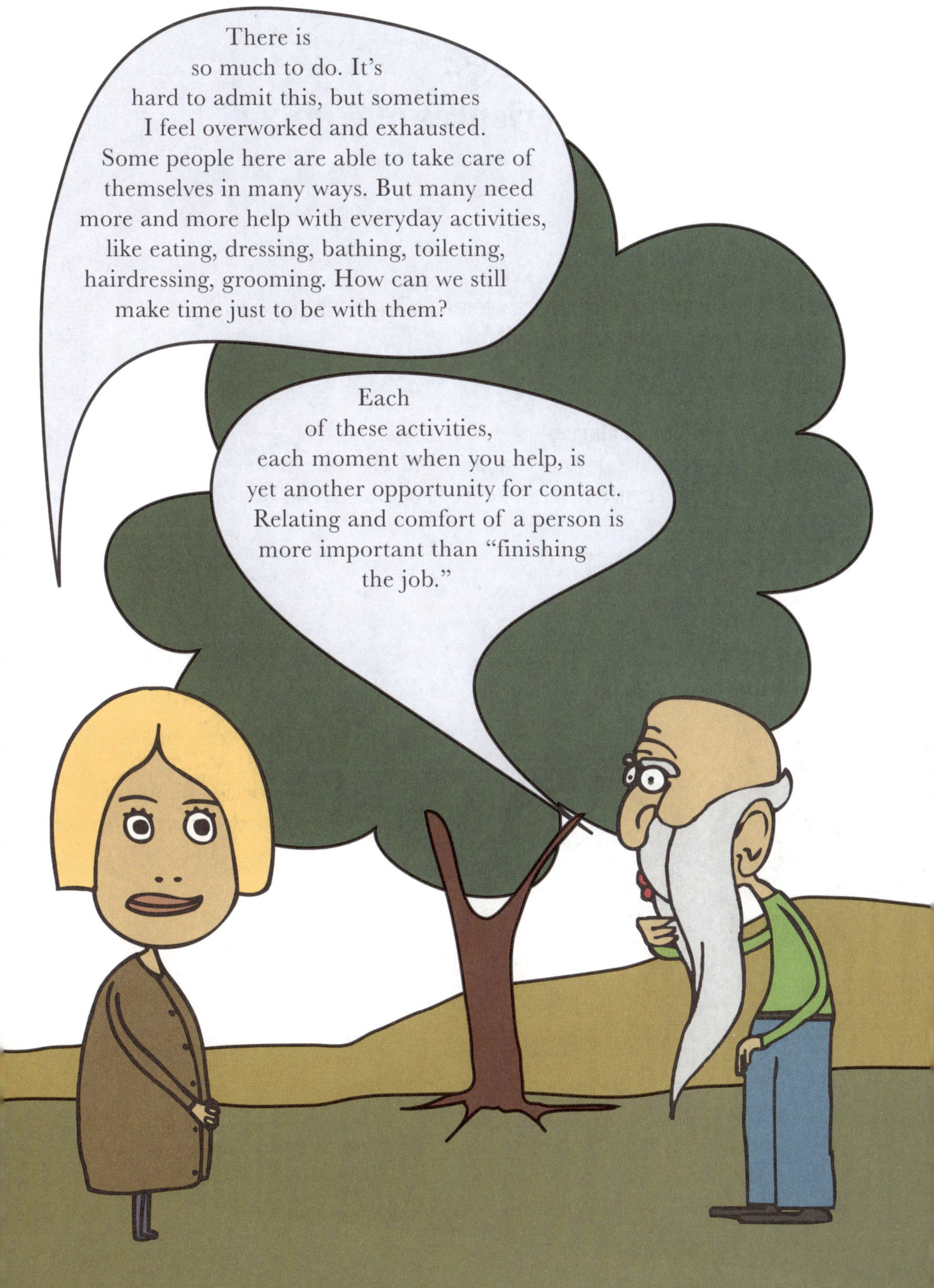
There is so much to do. It's hard to admit this, but sometimes I feel overworked and exhausted. Some people here are able to take care of themselves in many ways. But many need more and more help with everyday activities, like eating, dressing, bathing, toileting, hairdressing, grooming. How can we still make time just to be with them?
Each of these activities, each moment when you help, is yet another opportunity for contact. Relating and comfort of a person is more important than "finishing the job."

Daily Living Activities: Pleasurable Experiences of Contact

Dressing

Preparation:

- Adapt to a person's changing skills.
- Select clothing that is appropriate for the activities the person likes.
- Choose comfortable items.

Tips:

- Limit the number of choices.
- Organize the process: lay out clothing in the order the person will put it on.
- Give simple and concrete instructions: "Put this shirt on" rather than "Get dressed."
- Take one step at a time.
- Be flexible.
- Do not rush.
- Do not argue.

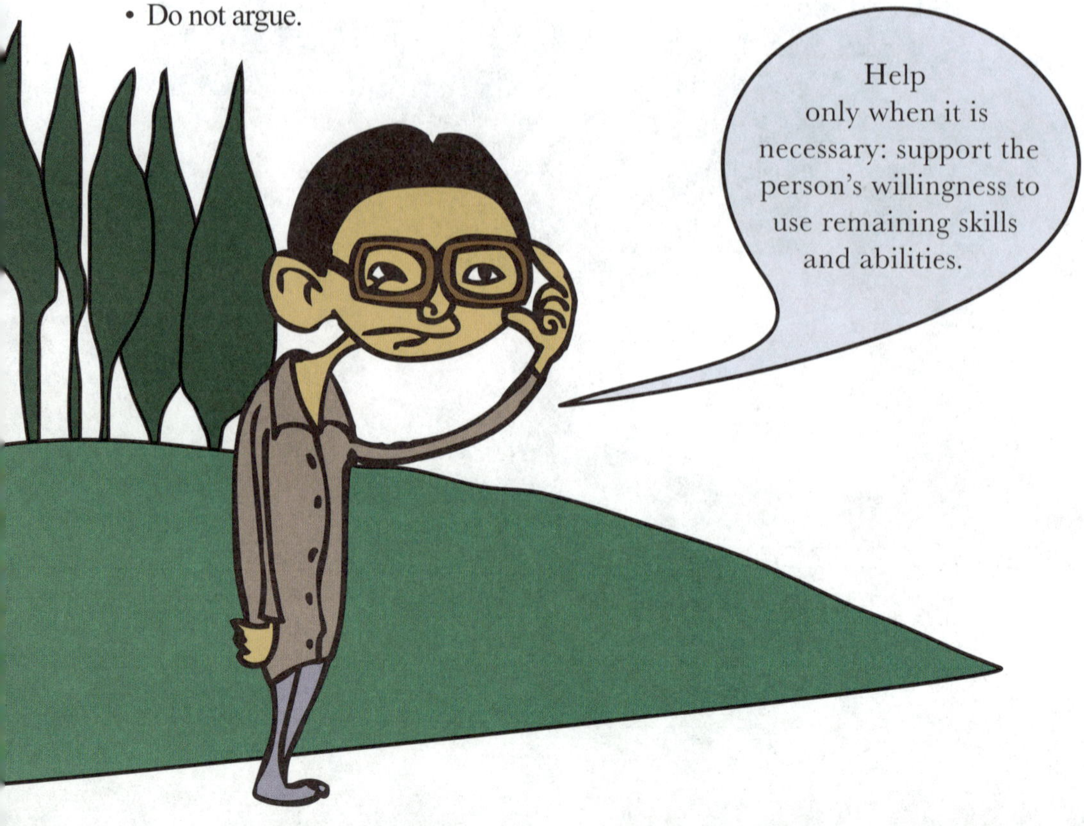
Help only when it is necessary: support the person's willingness to use remaining skills and abilities.

Bathing

Elderly may experience:
- Unpleasant sensations: cold, hot, pain.
- Fear of the unknown.
- Feeling of being dominated or insulted.
- Invasion of personal space.
- Misinterpreting caregiver behavior as harmful.
- Fear of spraying water.
- Loss of control.

Tips:
- Approach a person from the front.
- Tell the person what you are doing.
- Ask questions like: "Are you not used to undressing in front of other people? Did you ever undress in front of your sister or brother?"
- Provide privacy with extra towels.
- If a person is agitated, find another moment, or try a partial bath.
- Say "Thank you" or give a hug after finishing the task.

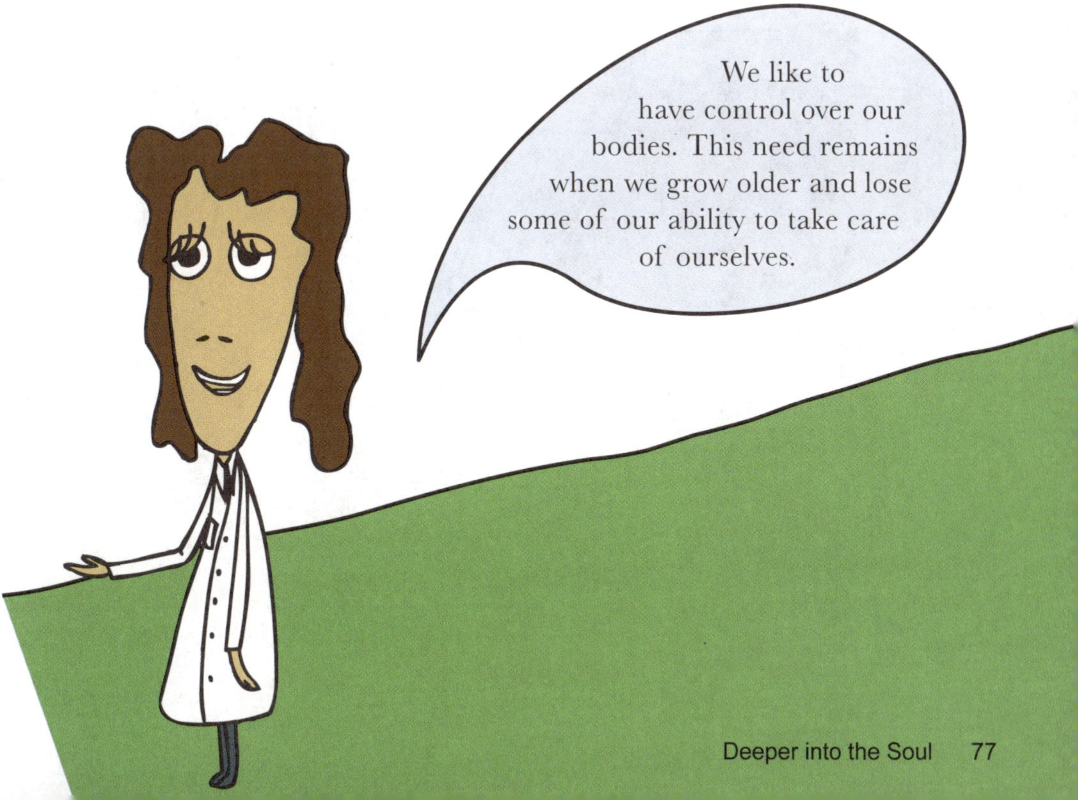
We like to have control over our bodies. This need remains when we grow older and lose some of our ability to take care of ourselves.

Toileting

Helping with incontinence:

- Stick to a toileting schedule.
- Monitor bowel movements and plan accordingly.
- Provide reminders.
- Look for cues indicating the person needs to use a bathroom.
- Make sure to report cases of incontinence and check for medical causes.
- Prevent dehydration; avoid diuretics (black tea, coffee, coke) and soda.

Tips:

- Help the person retain a sense of dignity.
- Respect privacy (look the other way if a person seems embarrassed).
- Don't punish or reproach inappropriate urination or other behaviors.

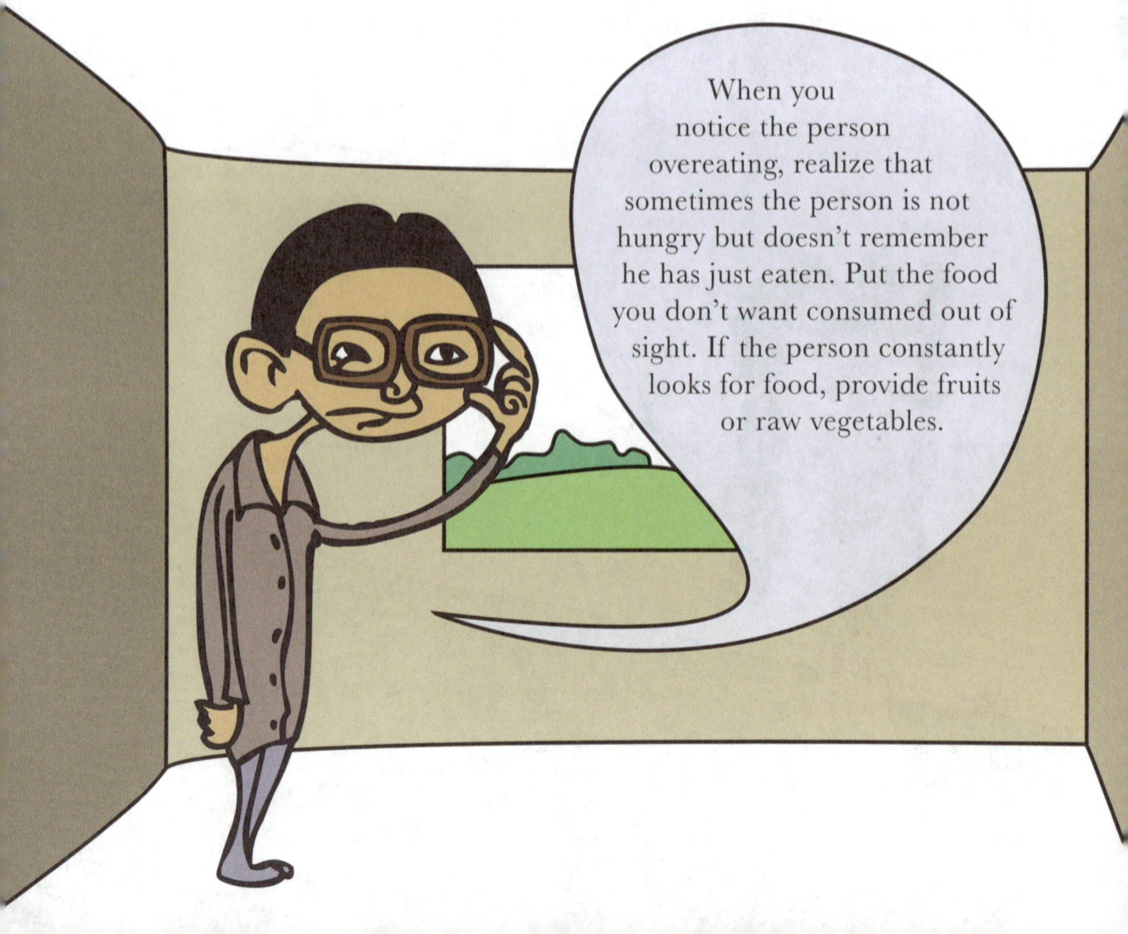
When you notice the person overeating, realize that sometimes the person is not hungry but doesn't remember he has just eaten. Put the food you don't want consumed out of sight. If the person constantly looks for food, provide fruits or raw vegetables.

Eating

Tips:

- Check the care plan for the person and stick to it.
- Keep in mind what helps the person and what is potentially harmful.
- Try to involve the person in the eating process: don't feed her if it is not necessary.
- If you must feed the person, try to put food into his hand and guide it to the mouth.
- Make eating a pleasant social experience.

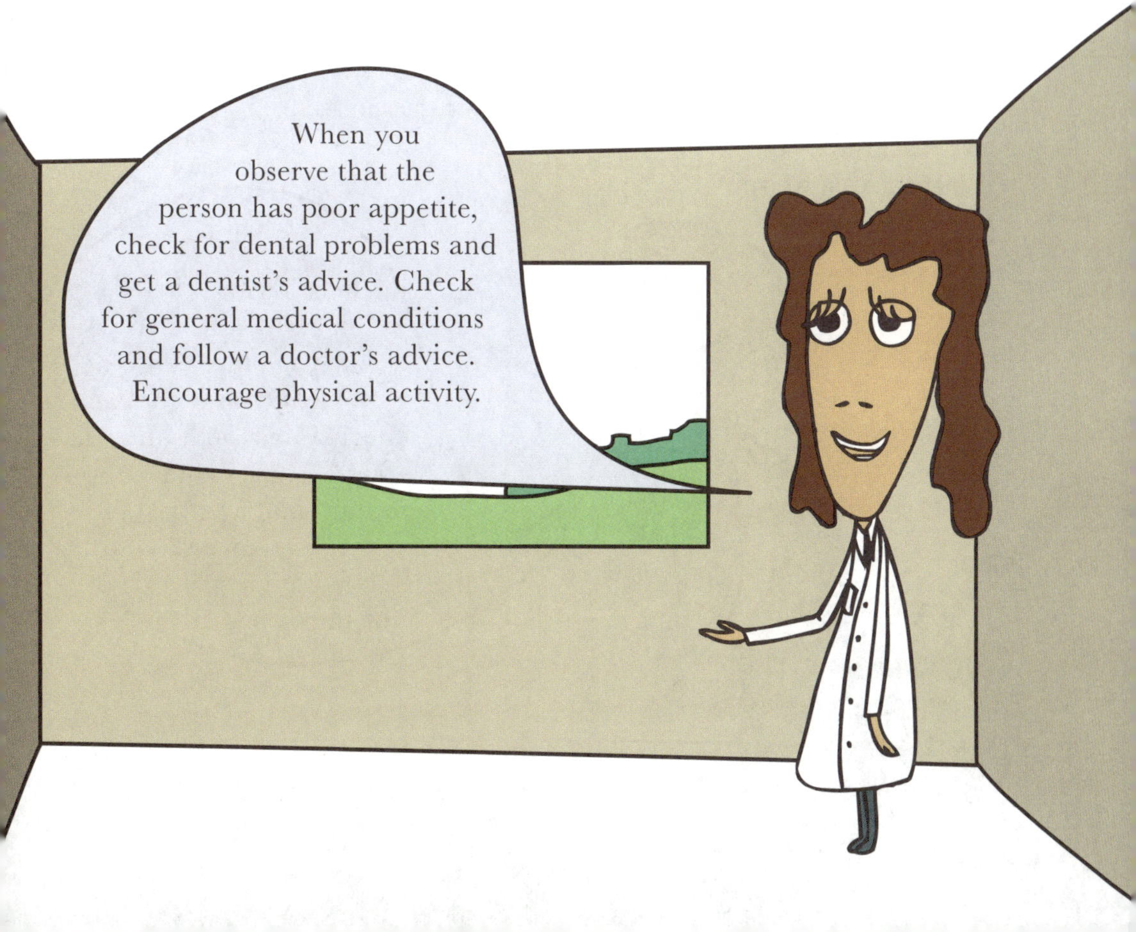
When you observe that the person has poor appetite, check for dental problems and get a dentist's advice. Check for general medical conditions and follow a doctor's advice. Encourage physical activity.

Challenging Behaviors

Some types of behavior are especially challenging to us. We get scared or simply don't understand. Yet it's important to consider that for people who act this way, it may be the best response to the situation they perceive. Imagine how you would feel if you were alone and afraid and misunderstood by everybody around you. Would you get angry? Cry?

Try to answer the following questions:

- WHEN does such behavior take place? (What time of the day? What kind of activity is occurring?)
- WHERE does it happen? (Evaluate the environment: number of people around, noise, lighting, stimulation level.)
- WHAT happened just before? (Did something trigger this behavior?)
- WHO may be involved? (Does the person react to people in the room? or perhaps to figures or memories from the past?)
- WHY does the person need to act in such a way? (What are the feelings and needs behind the behavior?)

To develop your best response, ask the following questions:

- What helps?
- What makes it worse?

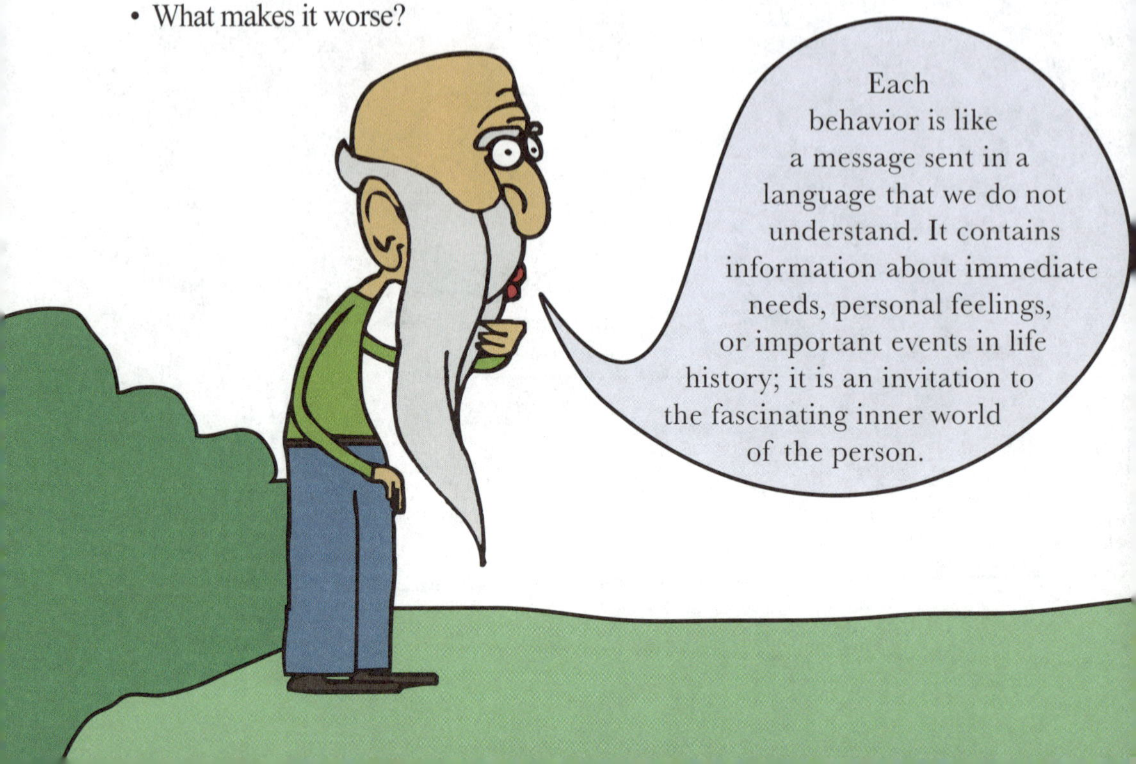
Each behavior is like a message sent in a language that we do not understand. It contains information about immediate needs, personal feelings, or important events in life history; it is an invitation to the fascinating inner world of the person.

Most Common Causes of Challenging Behaviors

Physical discomfort
Pain, fatigue, hunger, cold, bathroom needs, medication side effects.

Emotional discomfort
Loss of control, embarrassment, anxiety, loneliness, boredom.

Difficult social interactions
Inability to understand or express needs, difficulty recognizing people, feeling hurt by someone.

Sensory overload
Too much noise, too many people, overly complicated patterns.

Unfamiliar surrounding
Inability to recognize places and objects, difficulty finding one's way.

Complicated tasks
Difficulty with self-care, activities, and tasks.

Visions or voices from the inner world
Scary images, difficult or painful memories.

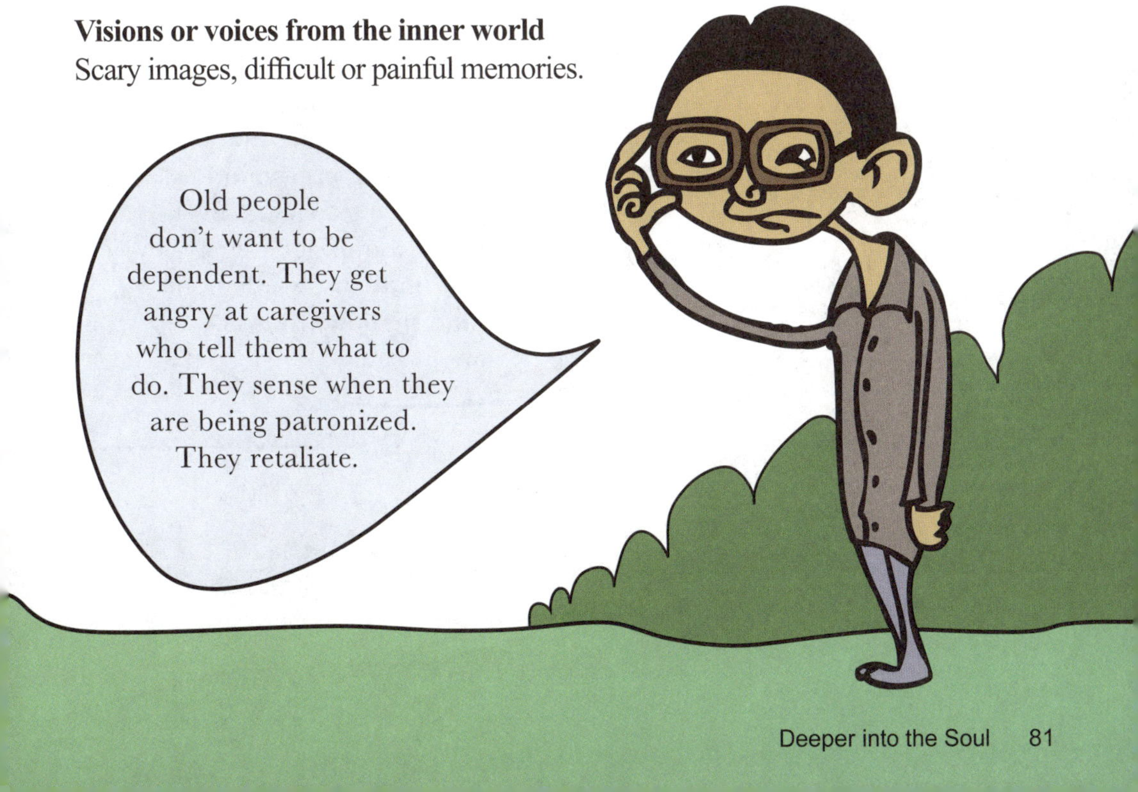
Old people don't want to be dependent. They get angry at caregivers who tell them what to do. They sense when they are being patronized. They retaliate.

Agitation and Aggression

Yes

- Respect personal space.
- Try to identify and remove immediate triggers.
- Acknowledge and help to express feelings:
  "No wonder you got furious!," "That made you angry!," "What was the worst thing that happened?"
- Listen to frustration: "Tell me more about this issue; you have good reason to be frustrated."
- Minimize distractions: turn the TV down (or off); avoid loud voices and commotion.

No

- Don't take things personally.
- Don't argue or reason.
- Don't tell the person to calm down before her frustration is expressed.
- Don't get upset.
- Avoid angry body language.
- Don't restrain the person unless there is immediate physical danger.

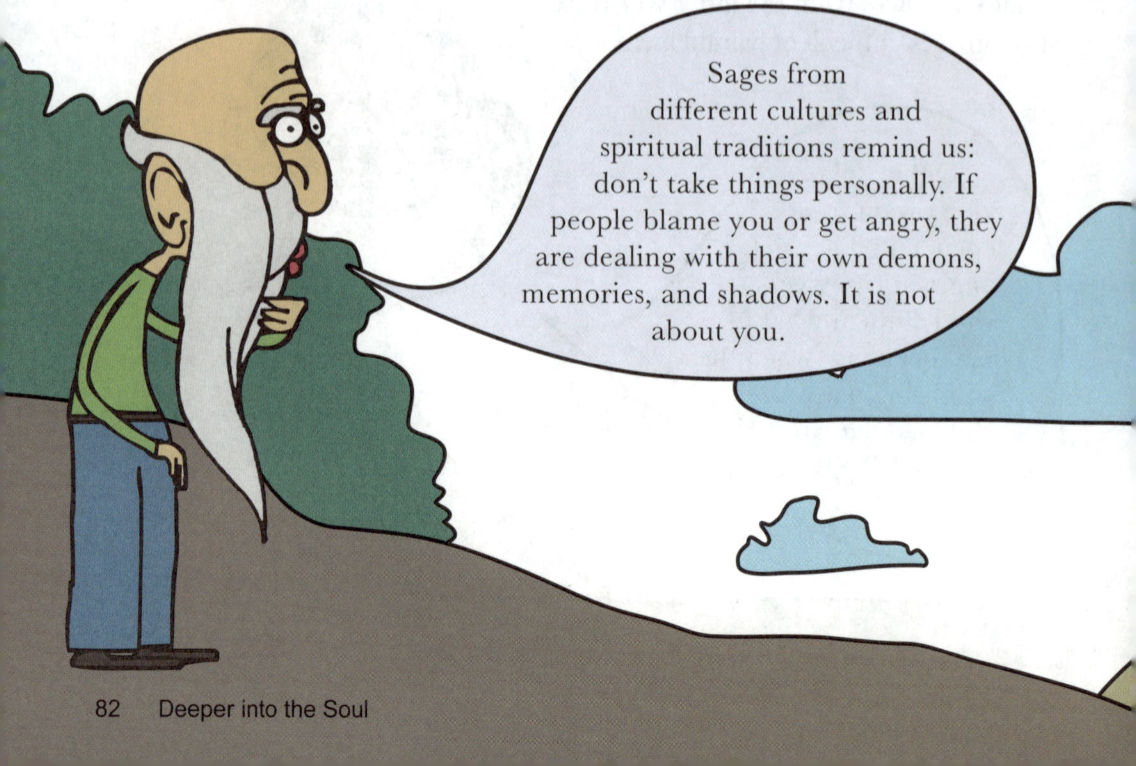
Sages from different cultures and spiritual traditions remind us: don't take things personally. If people blame you or get angry, they are dealing with their own demons, memories, and shadows. It is not about you.

Inappropriate Sexual Behavior

Yes

- Discourage sexual behavior in public.
- Lead person to his room; help find privacy.
- Involve person in structured activities.
- Redirect attention.
- Be gentle and firm.
- Check if the behavior is a result of confusion rather than sexual needs (getting into bed with another person, walking around undressed).

No

- Don't be confrontational.
- Avoid shaming or inflicting guilt.
- Don't get angry or upset.

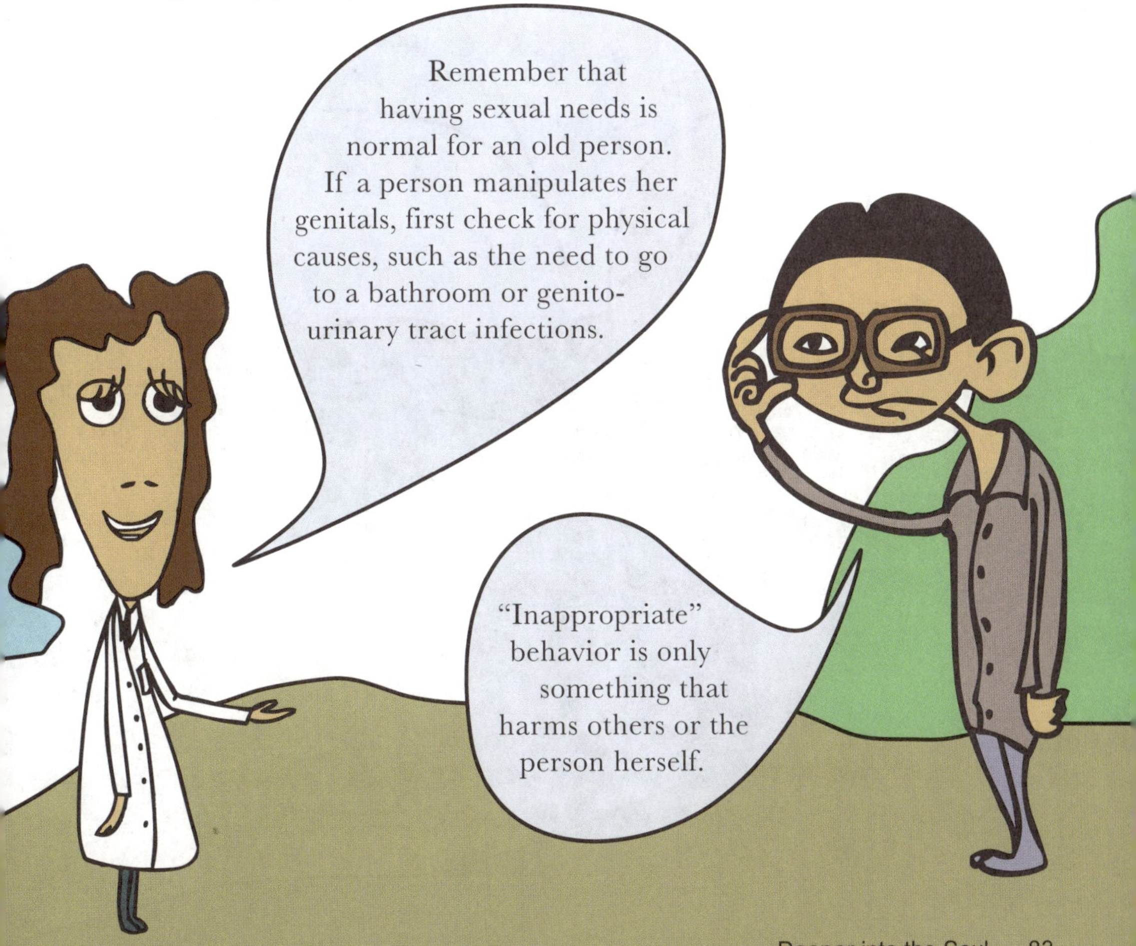
Remember that having sexual needs is normal for an old person. If a person manipulates her genitals, first check for physical causes, such as the need to go to a bathroom or genito-urinary tract infections.
"Inappropriate" behavior is only something that harms others or the person herself.

Screaming and Yelling

Yes

- Check for immediate triggers (pain, anxiety, boredom).
- Use calm, reassuring voice.
- Engage the person in other activities.
- Give a few minutes of undivided attention.
- Try to feel the same way the old person feels, and express his emotion with emotion: "You are so angry; did someone hurt you?"

No

- Don't get upset.
- Don't show your indifference.
- Don't treat the person like a child.

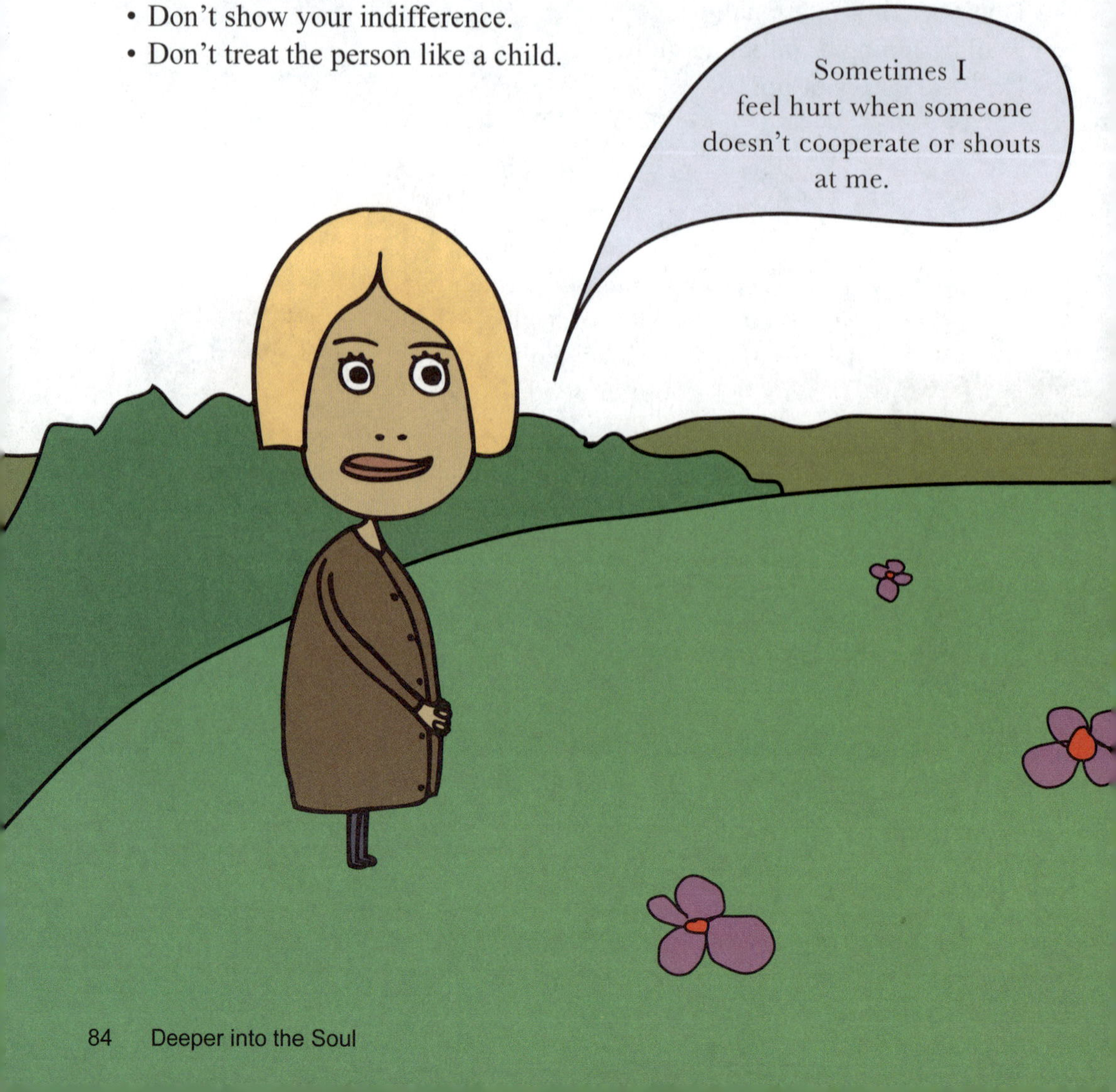
Sometimes I feel hurt when someone doesn't cooperate or shouts at me.

Wandering

Yes

- Check for physical discomfort.
- Find ways to use energy (regular exercise, walks).
- Engage the person in recreational activities.
- Try to find out if he is looking for something or someone from the past; help to express feelings.
- Make sure the environment is safe.
- Hide objects that may encourage wandering (coats, handbag).

No

- Don't reproach a person after she returns.
- Don't make sarcastic remarks.

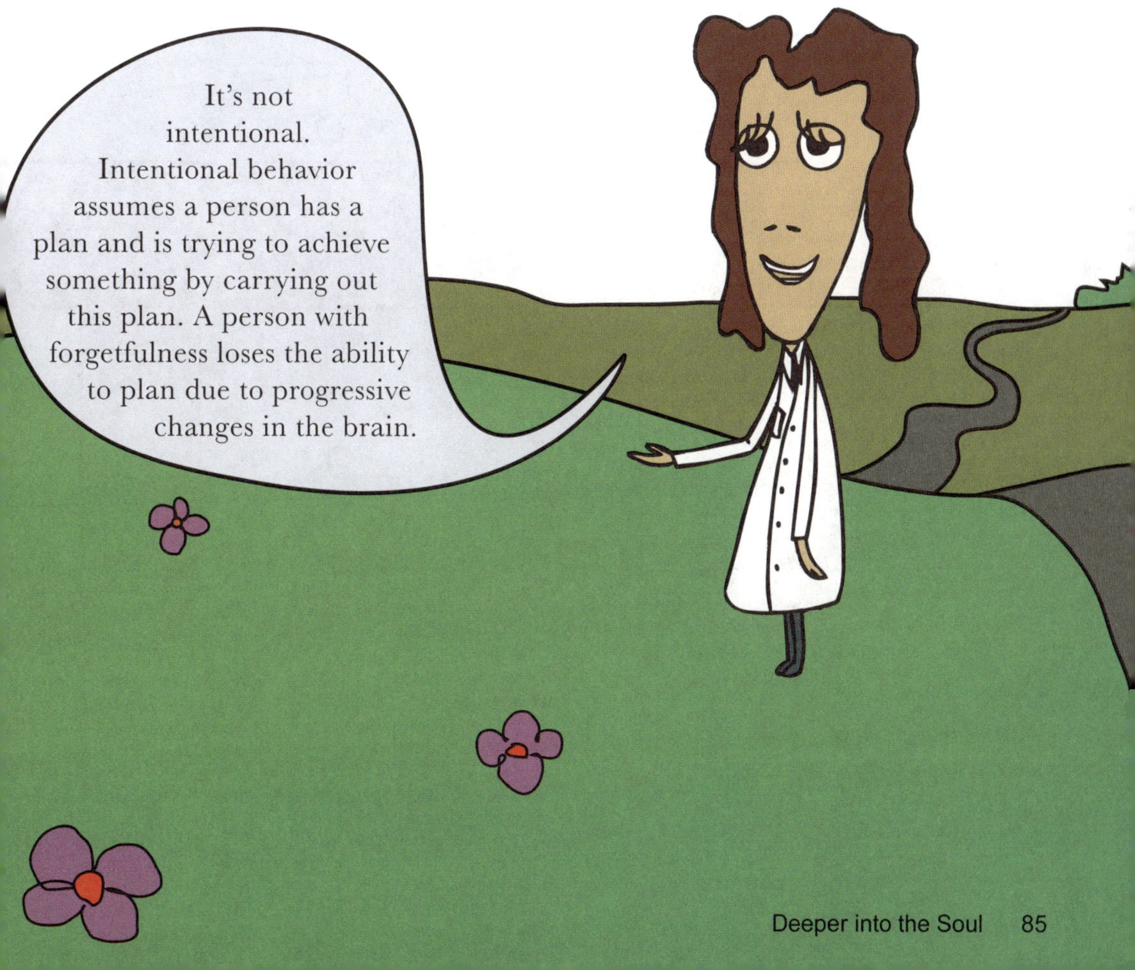
It's not intentional. Intentional behavior assumes a person has a plan and is trying to achieve something by carrying out this plan. A person with forgetfulness loses the ability to plan due to progressive changes in the brain.

Repetitive Motions: Pacing and Folding

Yes

- Remember that the person is trying to communicate; movements can replace speech.
- Try making movements together, such as moving your hands in the same way.
- Mirror body language.
- Acknowledge feelings.
- Accept the behavior and work with it; for example: if the person tries to fold his dirty tissue, give him some napkins to fold.
- Appreciate what she is doing and let her add her own meaning: "How nice that you have done…; thank you for doing…."

No

- Don't tell him to stop unless it is harmful.
- Don't restrain her movement.
- Don't ask him to explain what he is doing.

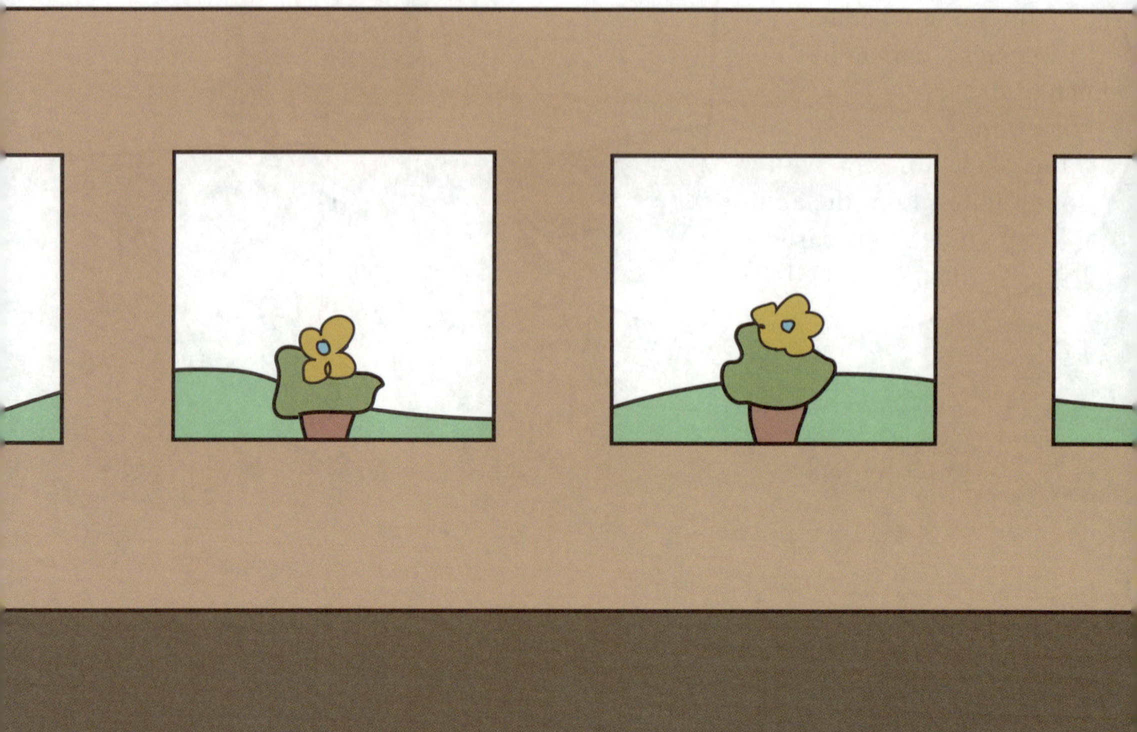

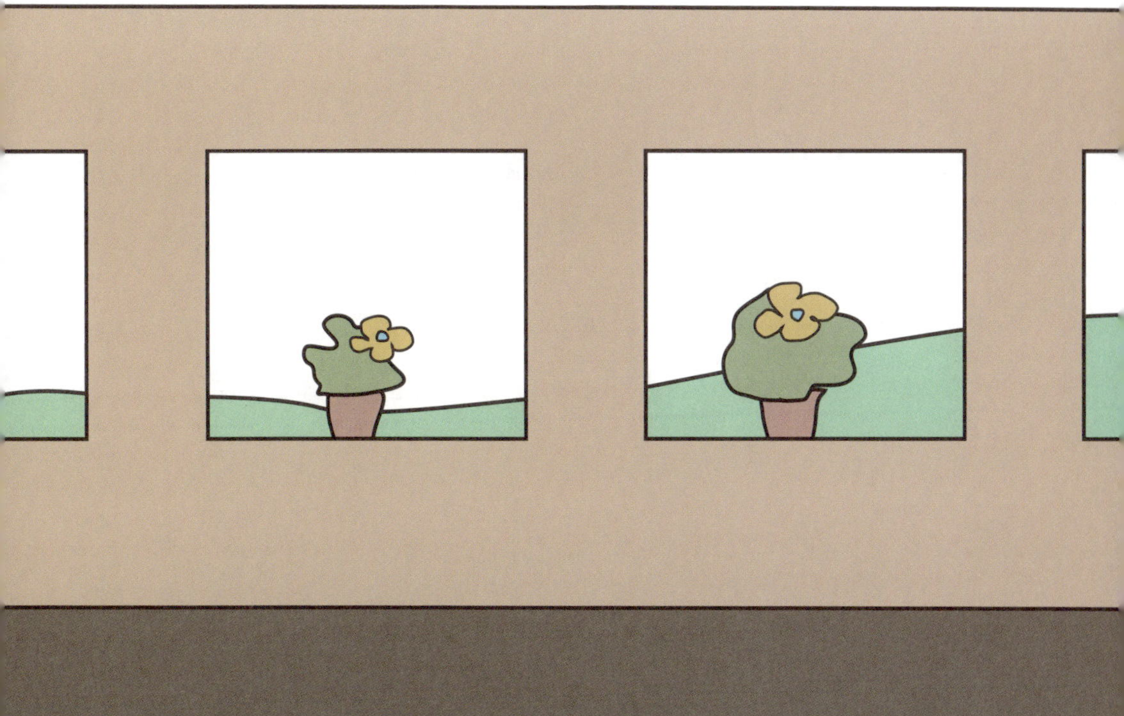

Through the symptom the psyche demands attention. Attention means attending to, tending, a certain tender care of, as well as waiting, pausing, listening. It takes a span of time and a tension of patience. Precisely what each symptom needs is time and tender care and attention. Just this same attitude is what the soul needs in order to be felt and heard.

— *James Hillman*

Appendix

Inspiration from Different Approaches

Forgetfulness Care as a Meta-Perspective

Forgetfulness care, as described in this book, serves as a general perspective. It helps us look at the phenomenon called dementia with compassion, curiosity, and openness. It allows us to embrace different information, techniques, and methods. We have been inspired by various approaches that have been developed over the past few decades. Here we present some of those approaches.

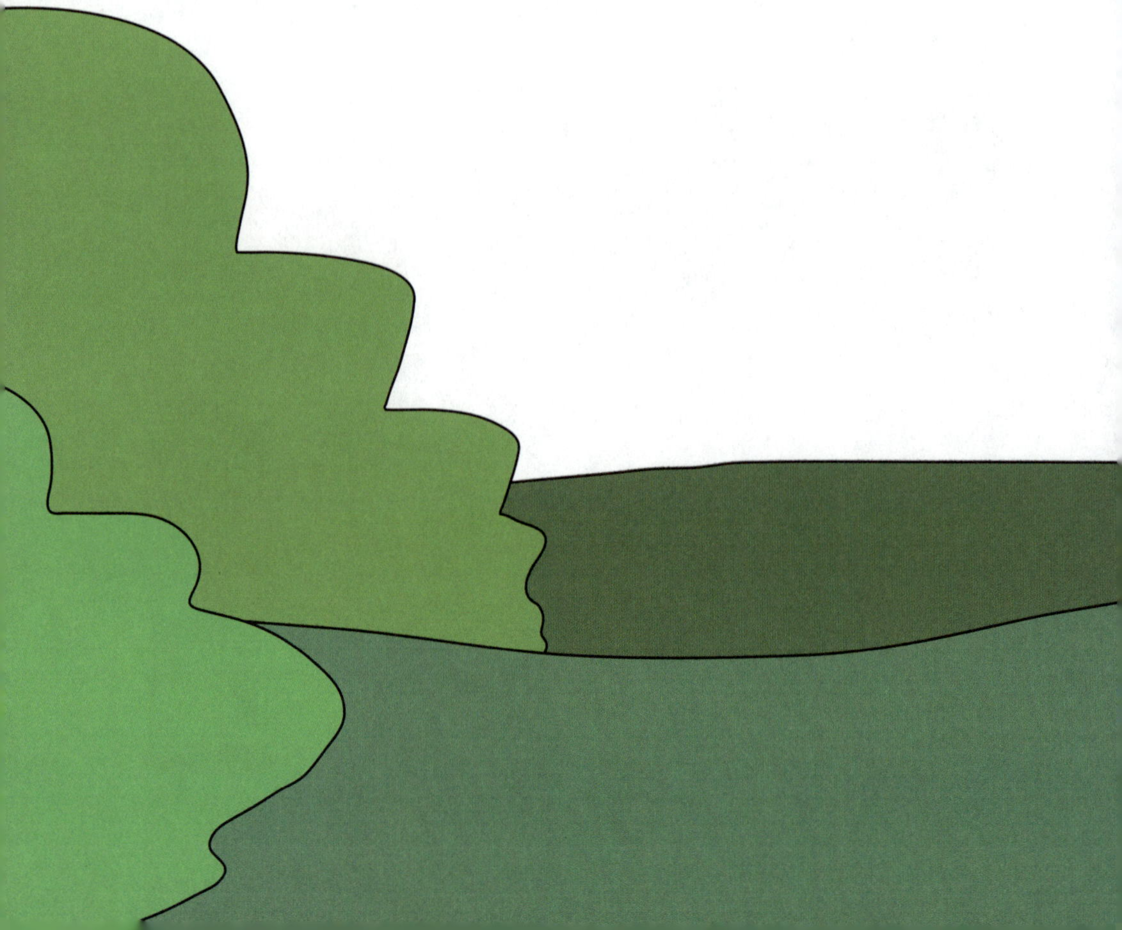

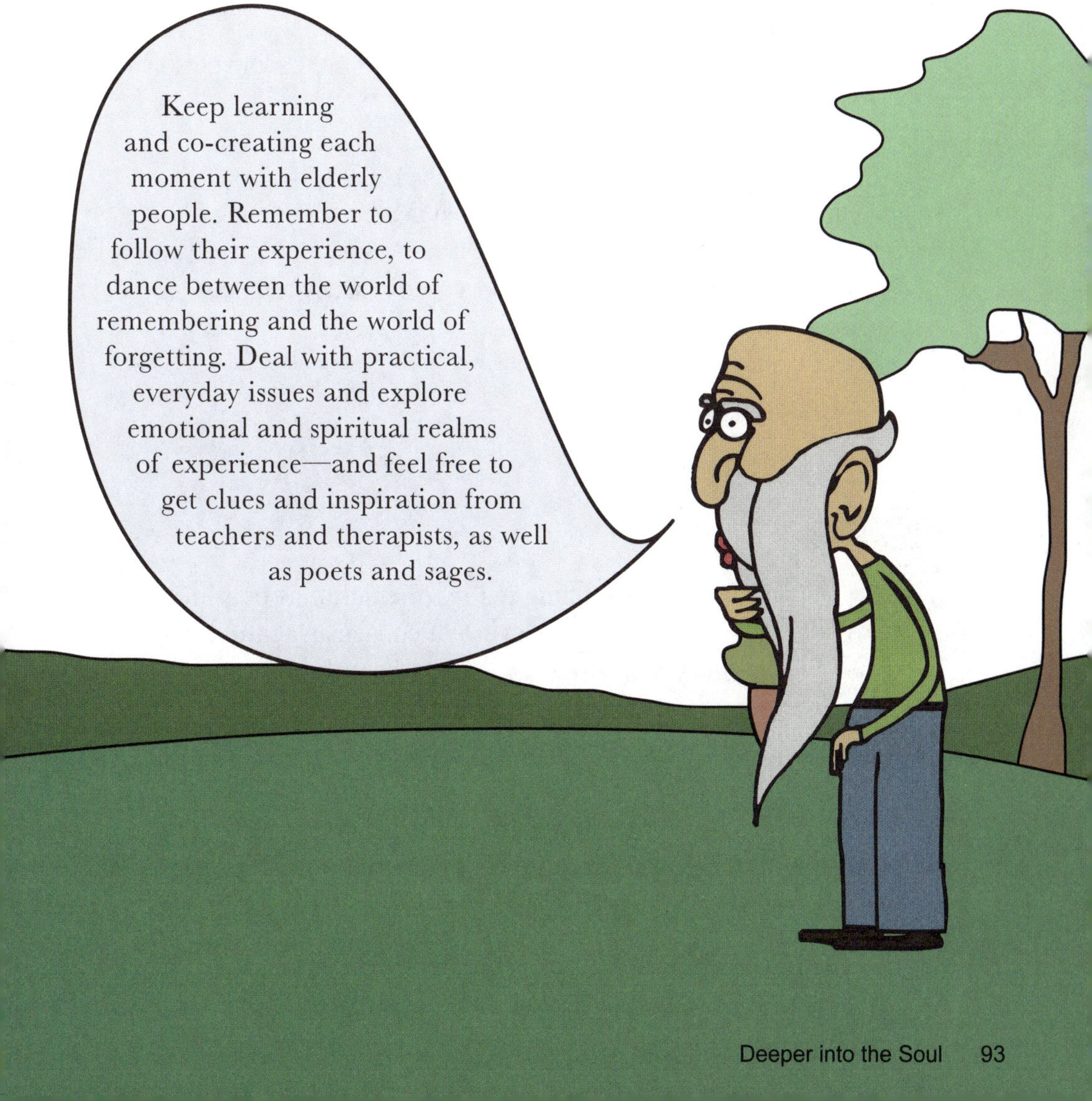
Keep learning and co-creating each moment with elderly people. Remember to follow their experience, to dance between the world of remembering and the world of forgetting. Deal with practical, everyday issues and explore emotional and spiritual realms of experience—and feel free to get clues and inspiration from teachers and therapists, as well as poets and sages.

Reality Orientation

Goals and assumptions:

- Reality orientation is a set of techniques that helps a person with forgetfulness feel more at home in our consensus reality.
- It consists of repeated cues and guidelines that lessen confusion and facilitate orientation in this reality.
- It aims to help the person feel more independent, more confident, with higher self-esteem.

Techniques:

- Friendly attitude toward patients.
- Repeated presentation of basic orienting information:
  - Visual cues: clocks; boards with date, time, month, season; personal items and photos.
  - Reminding a person who she is.
  - Stating your name when you approach the person.
- Helping the elderly be interested and involved in their environment.
  - Organizing activities.
  - Encouraging them to notice and take care of the environment (places, animals, plants).
  - Social contacts.

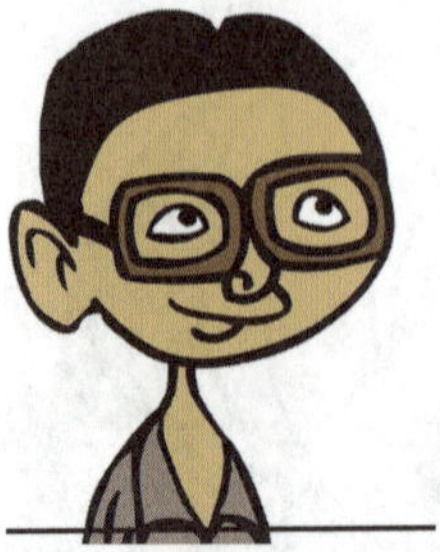

Non-patronizing reality orientation is helpful for people who are aware of consensus reality; who forget and want to know where they are.

Memory Training

Goals:

Memory training focuses on cognitive functioning, mainly remembering and retrieving information from memory.

Techniques:

- Procedures carefully chosen to support self-confidence—otherwise it may be frustrating and anxiety raising.
- Specially developed procedures (games, exercises) to help the person learn new material and to recall it.

Reality Orientation Board Example

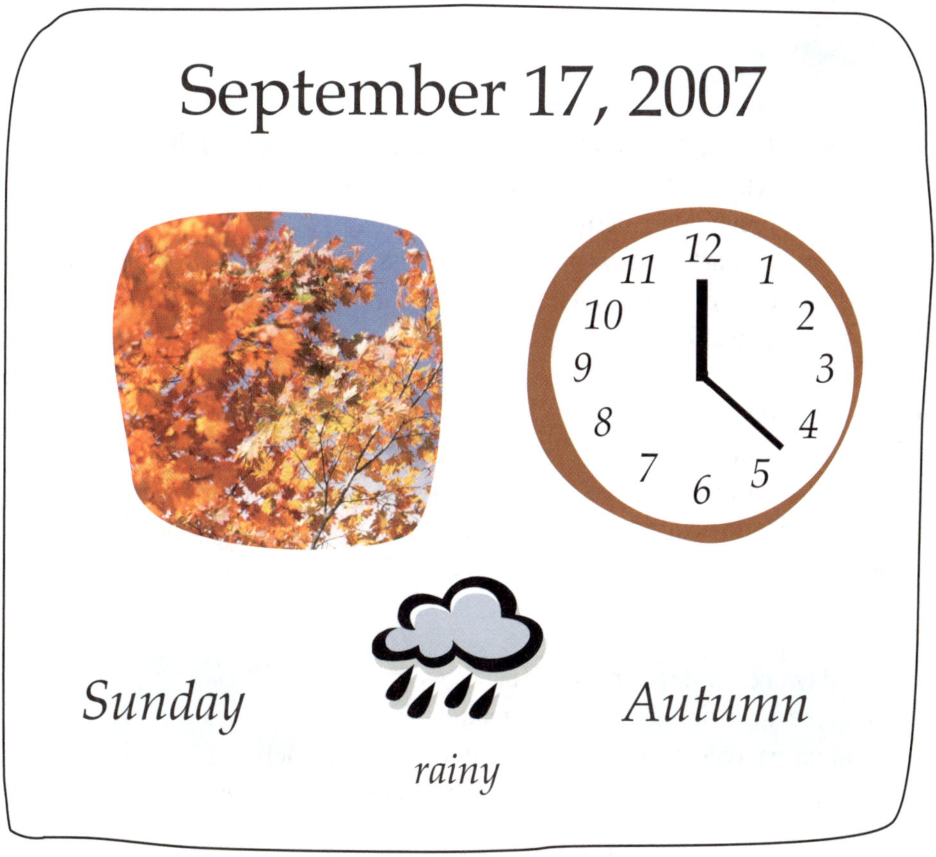

Reminiscence Therapy

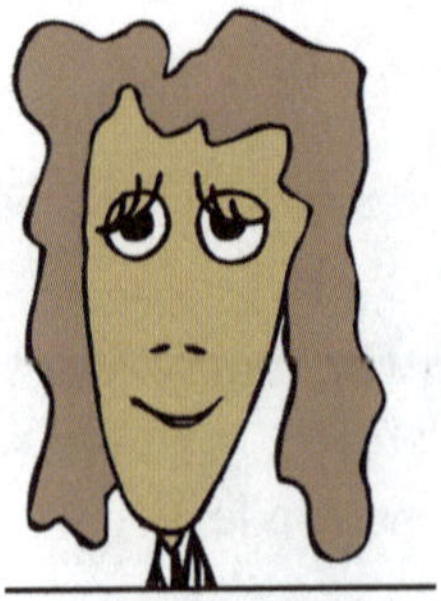

Robert Butler, pioneer reminiscence therapist, recalls that in the 1950s "living in the past" was seen as a symptom of senility, as one of the signs of living a meaningless life.

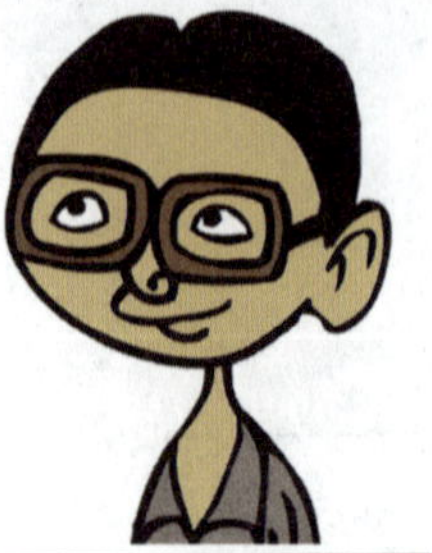

In a recent article Butler writes, "Far from living in the past or exhibiting 'wandering of the mind,' as was commonly thought, older people are engaged in the important psychological tasks of making sense of the lives they had lived."

Goals and assumptions:

- Old people try to understand who they are and the meaning of their life by reconstructing their memories and telling stories from the past.
- They often retain vivid memories.
- They work on past conflicts and unfinished issues by talking about their memories.
- The purpose of remembering and reconstructing the past and telling stories is to find the meaning in one's life journey.

Types of reminiscence

- Simple storytelling.
- Looking at past events from a new point of view.
- Dealing with difficult emotional issues from the past on both a literal and metaphoric level.

Techniques

- Everyday one-on-one conversations.
- Group meetings and directed storytelling.
- Use of props: objects from the past, photos, music, smells.
- Use of art to capture meaning beyond the literal sense of the story.

Habilitation Therapy

Goals and assumptions

Alzheimer's disease was once seen as:

- A "normal part of aging," which led to the notion that no treatment is needed.
- A "low-tech area of medicine" where only basic care is needed.
- A fatal condition that should be cured through biomedical means, with a focus on medical research.

In contrast, the authors of habilitation therapy understand forgetfulness as a disability. They assume that:

- Coping with a disability depends largely on environmental factors.
- It is helpful to focus on remaining capacities rather than on what is lost.
- The main aim is not rehabilitation, in the sense of restoring previous abilities of people with forgetfulness, but to help them to maximize their independent functioning and to feel good about themselves in their present condition.

Techniques:

- Organizing the environment in a way that provides comfort and clear orienting cues.
- Encouraging participation in structured social activities that do not lead to a sense of failure.
- Helping to use remaining functions in daily life.
- Appropriate nonverbal communication focused on feelings.
- Understanding the differences in perception.
- Responding to challenging behavior by positive problem-solving.

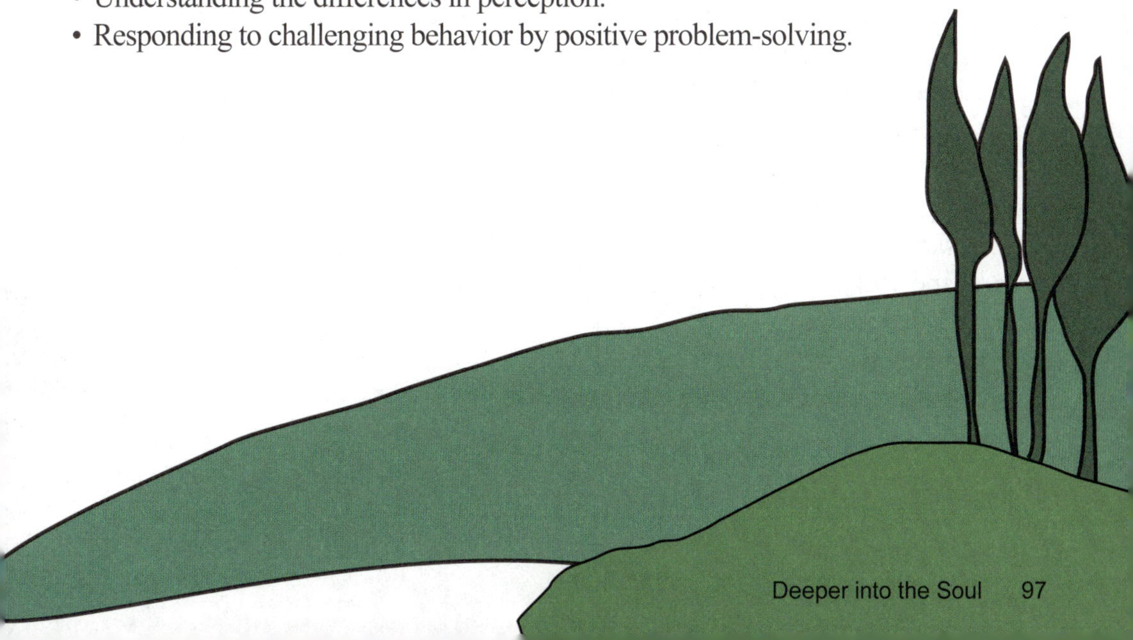

Validation Therapy

Painful feelings that are expressed, acknowledged, and validated by a trusted listener will diminish. Painful feelings that are ignored or suppressed will gain strength and can become toxic.

—Naomi Feil, *Validation Breakthrough*

Goals and assumptions

- Validation therapy has been developed by Naomi Feil from the 1960s to the present.
- Old age is understood as yet another important phase in life: the resolution phase.
- The main task in this phase is to resolve inner conflicts and emotional issues from the past.
- Validation method is a practical way to communicate with old people that helps them express and get acknowledgment for their feelings.

Four stages of resolution

- Mal-orientation: People express past conflict or issues in a disguised form, confusing them with present events. They use present reality to get in touch with feelings (past and present) that they need to express but cannot do so directly.
- Time-confusion: People tend to withdraw more into their inner world, feeling lonely and abandoned in consensus reality. They need to get in touch with their feelings and need acceptance from others.
- Repetitive motion: People access and express their experiences through movement rather than words.
- Vegetation: People abandon the effort to resolve past issues.

Attitudes

- Respectful.
- Nonjudgmental.
- Empathetic.
- Focus on acknowledging feelings.

Techniques

- Different communication techniques are used at different stages.
- Validation can be used in one-on-one conversation or in a group setting.
- Basic communication guidelines are as follows:
    - Listen empathetically without judging.
    - Establish warm emotional contact through loving touch, eye contact, low and calm tone of voice.
    - Observe and match emotions.
    - Help the person express emotions by encouraging him to complete his story.
    - Ask factual questions.
    - Paraphrase answers—repeat in different words.
    - Communicate through movement—do it together.

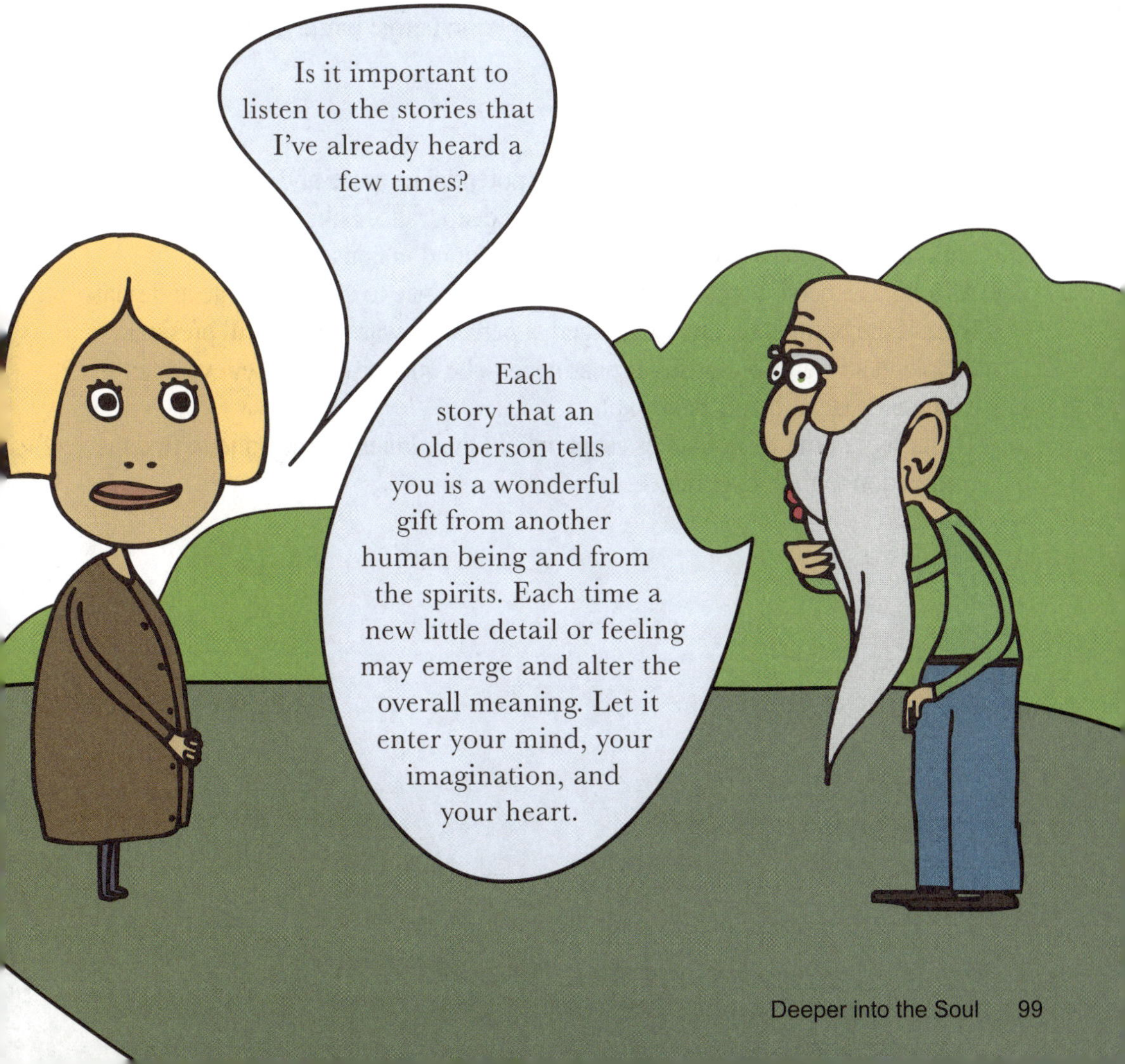
Is it important to listen to the stories that I've already heard a few times?
Each story that an old person tells you is a wonderful gift from another human being and from the spirits. Each time a new little detail or feeling may emerge and alter the overall meaning. Let it enter your mind, your imagination, and your heart.

Coma Work

Coma work is based on the philosophy that the human being in coma is on an inner journey. ... Therefore our effort is devoted to meeting individuals where they are, in that deepest, almost unfathomable, altered state of consciousness.

—Amy Mindell, *Coma: A Healing Journey*

Coma and other remote altered states

People with advanced forgetfulness often go back and forth between deep trance and closer contact to consensus reality. Even in long-term, so-called vegetative states, a part of the psyche keeps searching for contact, love, and meaning. Besides dealing with unresolved issues from their personal history, people in comas and advanced dementia wage metaphoric heroic battles and have strong spiritual experiences.

Goals and assumptions

- Each symptom, even a painful one, has potential purpose and meaning.
- Altered states of consciousness, including deep trances like coma, contain important information that often cannot be found in consensus reality.
- As long as a person is breathing, you have a chance to communicate and relate.
- Even if the brain is severely damaged, a person's awareness is still present.
- People in all states of consciousness need to be encouraged to believe that their experience is valid and important.
- The aim of coma work is to assist people in their inner journey and to find the completion to their experience.

Techniques

- Join a person through the rate of her breathing.
- Notice minimal signals: movement, sounds, skin-color changes.
- Mention the importance of such signals to the person for whom you are caring.
- Validate importance of the inner experience (even though you don't know the content). For example: "Follow what is happening inside of you"; "Trust your own experience."
- Notice the person's feedback: changes in skin color or breath, sounds, and movements in response to our interventions usually indicate positive feedback.
- Establish binary communication: choose a signal for "yes" and "no," and try to ask simple, answerable questions.
- Always treat a person in a coma or other deep trance with respect.

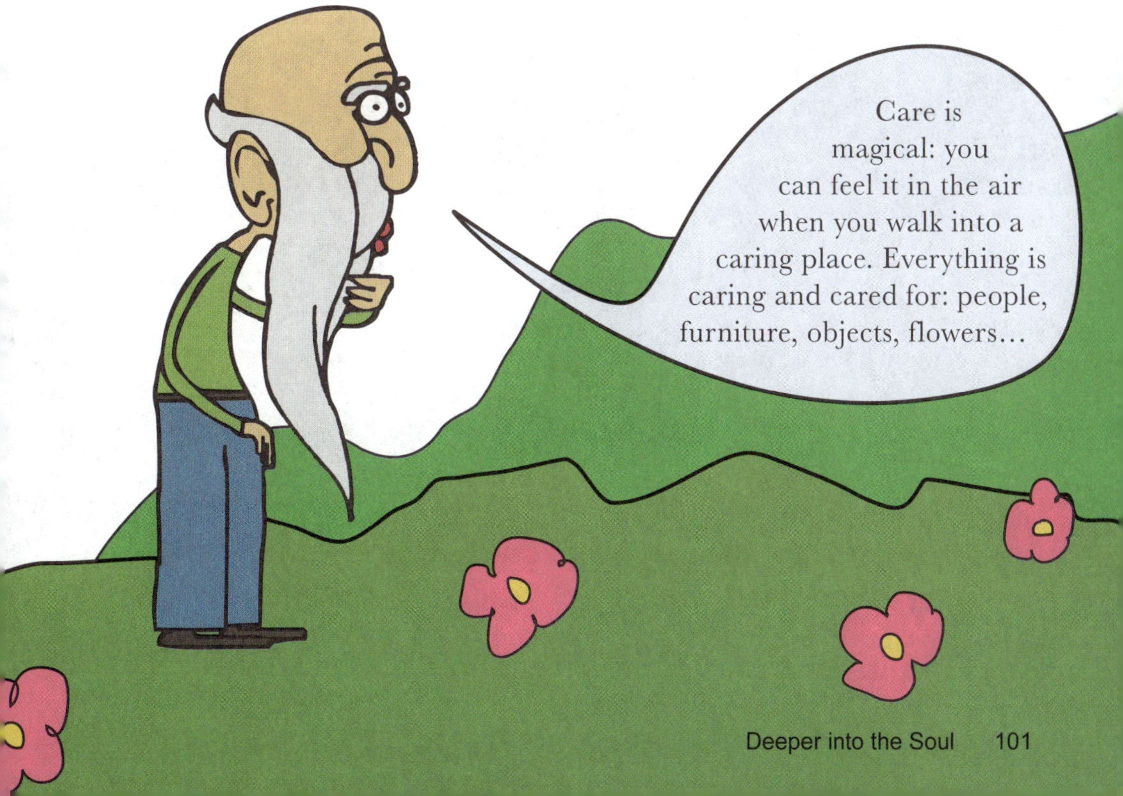
Care is magical: you can feel it in the air when you walk into a caring place. Everything is caring and cared for: people, furniture, objects, flowers…

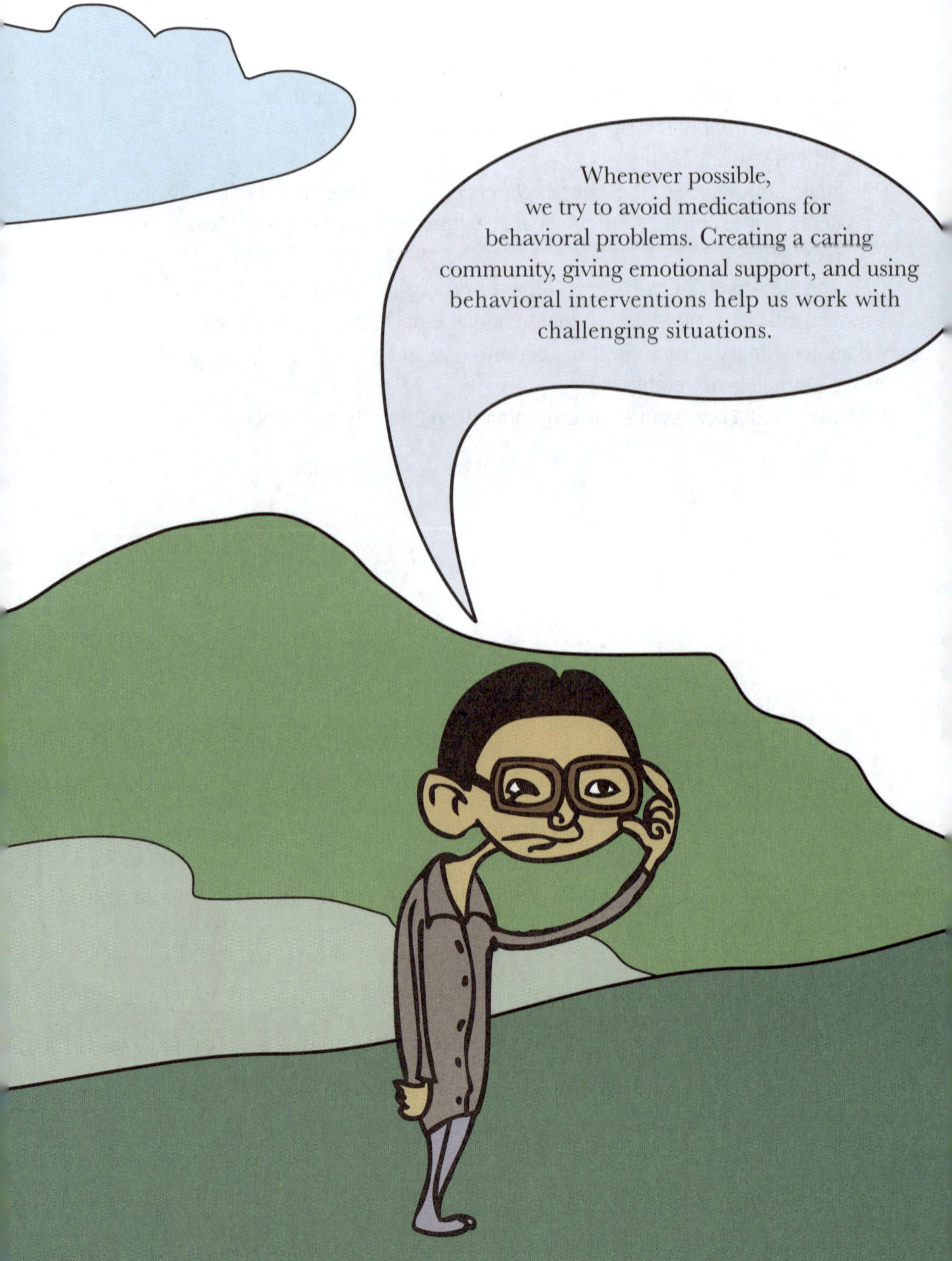
Whenever possible,
we try to avoid medications for
behavioral problems. Creating a caring
community, giving emotional support, and using
behavioral interventions help us work with
challenging situations.

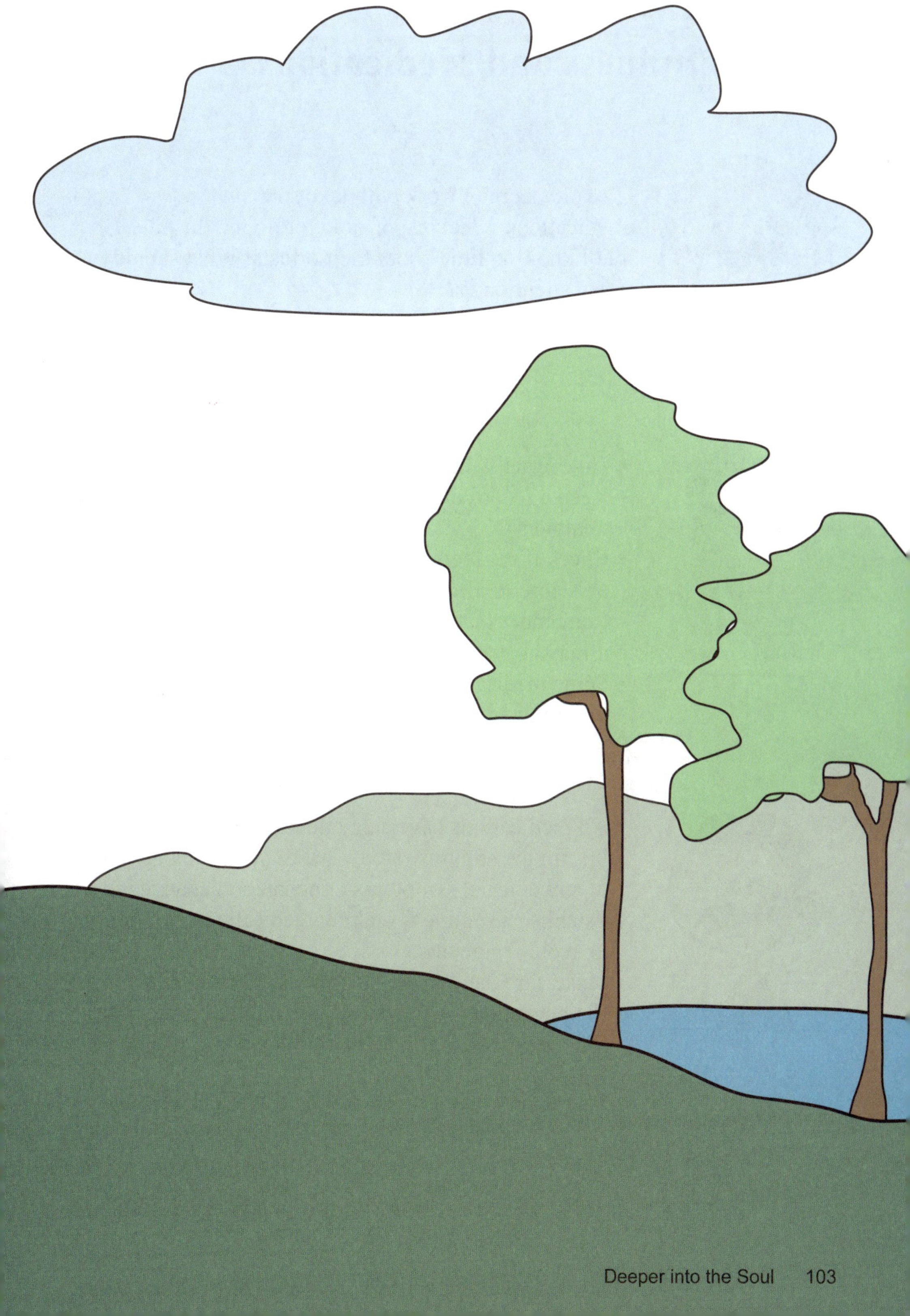

Forgetfulness and Medications

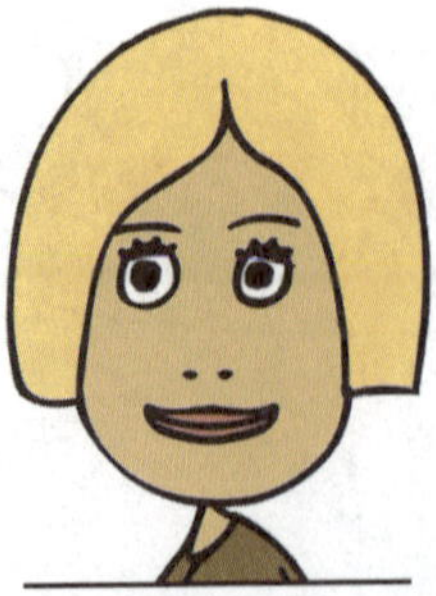

The old people I work with take so many medications. I feel responsible for giving the pills, but I know so little about their effects! What should I pay attention to?

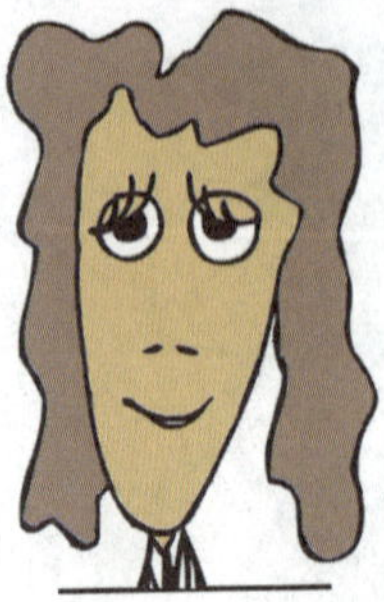

- Give exactly the prescribed dose at the given time of day.
- Keep a record of all medications (including alternative treatment).
- Check if the medication should be taken with food or before or after meals.
- Remember that not all medications work immediately; it may take a few weeks before you see the effects.
- Some medications that help at the early stage of forgetfulness are not effective in later phases.

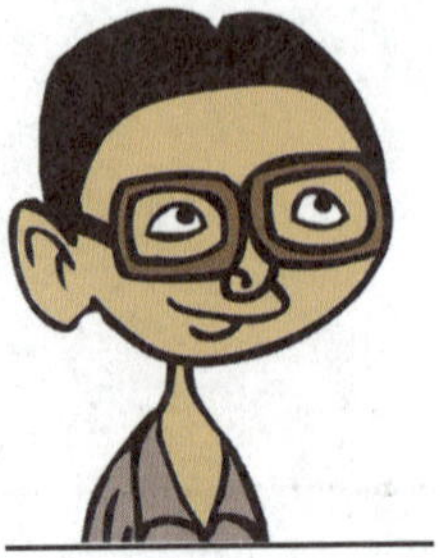

- All medications have side effects.
- Inform the administrative staff or doctor immediately of any unusual symptoms or behavioral changes.
- Establish a routine for taking medications; it helps to avoid arguments.
- Make sure that the medication has been swallowed.
- If a person has problems swallowing pills, ask if the same medications come in liquid form.

Treatment for Forgetfulness

Acetylcholinesterase (AChE) inhibitors

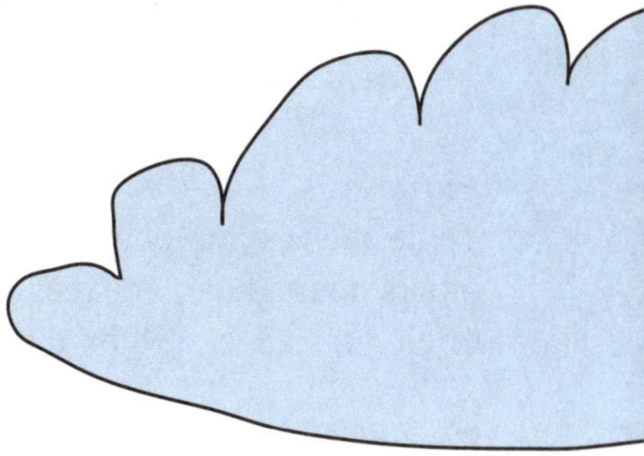

How they work:
Acetylcholine helps brain cells communicate. Medications prevent acetylocholine from breaking down in the brain.

Possible side effects:
Nausea, vomiting, headaches, dizziness, loss of appetite, muscle cramps, skin changes.

N-methyl D-aspartate (NMDA) blockers

How they work:
Malfunction of NMDA receptors in certain nerve cells causes overstimulation of these cells. As a result, these cells get damaged and die. NMDA blockers prevent the overstimulation of brain cells.

Possible side effects:
Dizziness, headaches, constipation.

Medications Used to Ease Behavioral Problems

Antipsychotics

Purpose:
To decrease symptoms such as otherworldly visions, hearing voices that others do not hear, or excessive suspiciousness. Agitation or aggression is often reduced as well by these medications.

Possible side effects:
Drowsiness, dizziness, increased sensitivity to light, weight gain, dry mouth, difficulty urinating, constipation, drooling, headaches.

Anti-anxiety drugs

Purpose:
To reduce anxiety or agitation; to help people suffering from insomnia (disorders of initiating and maintaining sleep).

Possible side effects:
Dizziness, fatigue, drowsiness, oversedation, depression, light-headedness, irritability, breathing problems. If used for longer periods of time, the medication may alter sleep patterns.

Antidepressants

Caution
Symptoms of depression may mask other physical conditions.

Purpose:
To reduce depressive symptoms, to improve mood, increase energy and appetite.

Possible side effects:
Nausea, vomiting, diarrhea, headaches and insomnia.

Mood stabilizers

Purpose:
To reduce fluctuations between manic and depressive moods.

Possible side effects:
Nausea, vomiting, sedation, gastric problems.

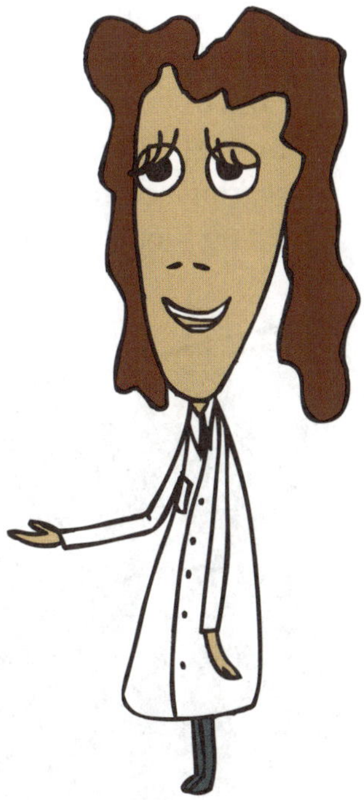

Being with Bereavement and Loss

"Let's hurry up to love people, they leave so quickly…"
—Jan Twardowski, poet and priest

Feelings of Loss

If you feel close to a person who develops symptoms of forgetfulness, you are likely to experience feelings of grief and loss—not only after a person dies, but also as the condition progresses.

This is sometimes called *anticipatory grief* and includes:
- Loss of a person you knew before.
- Loss of a relationship you liked.
- Loss of a person's former self.

Friends and family members may experience:
- Loss of future plans (going for holidays next year, taking care of the garden together).
- Loss of companionship and support.
- Loss of a lifestyle they once had together (reading newspapers and sharing comments every morning, going to the opera once a month, eating lunch at the kitchen table).

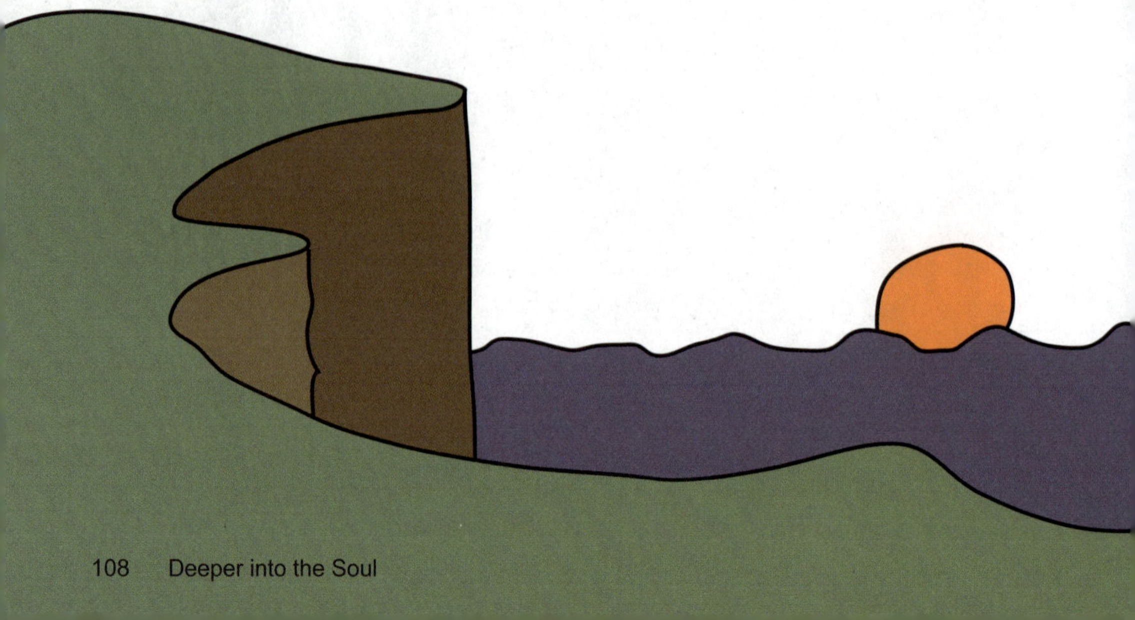

Caregivers may experience:
- Grief and a sense of loss when they see pain and suffering on a daily basis.
- Sadness and anger as a person with forgetfulness symptoms slowly goes to another realm.

Grieving for a person with forgetfulness symptoms alternates:
- Between despair and strong hope that everything will return to the way it was.
- Between acceptance and non-acceptance.

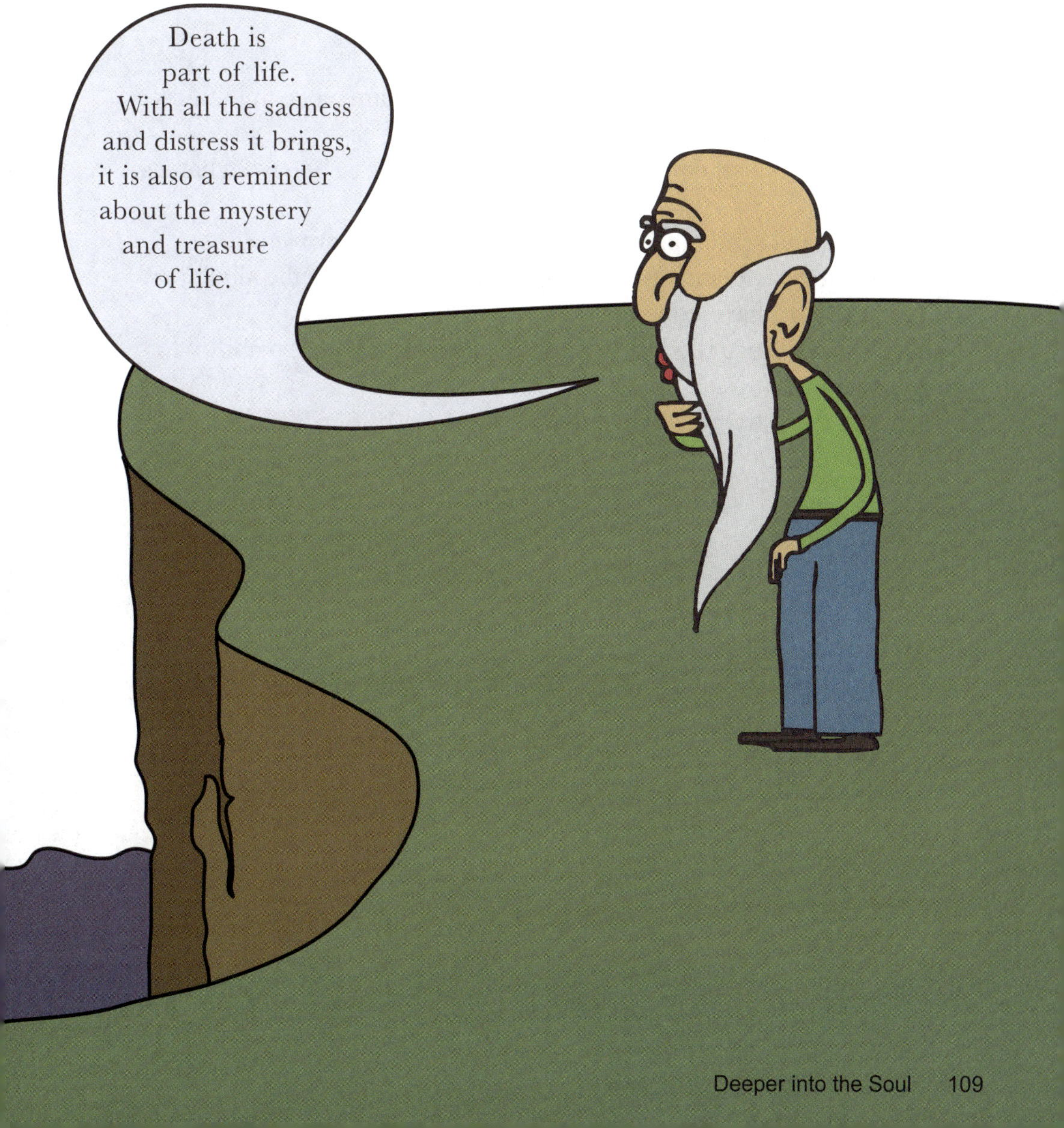
Death is part of life. With all the sadness and distress it brings, it is also a reminder about the mystery and treasure of life.

Death and Bereavement

> *"As caregivers, we are acutely aware of the fragility of life and the inevitability of death. Each day, we are called upon to facilitate healing and accompany others on their journeys. However, we rarely give ourselves space to breathe deeply and integrate the intensity of our experiences at the bedside."*
>
> —comment from Zen Hospice Project, National Nurses Week celebration

Reactions to Death

Common reactions to the death of a person you are close to include:

- Shock, numbness, emotional paralysis, inability to believe what has happened.
- Yearning and searching, denial mixed with strong anxiety.
- Bargaining with God, guilt, thoughts about reversing the situation (what could I have done better?).
- Depression, frustration, hopelessness, disorganization, inability to return to usual activities.
- Acceptance, coping with change.

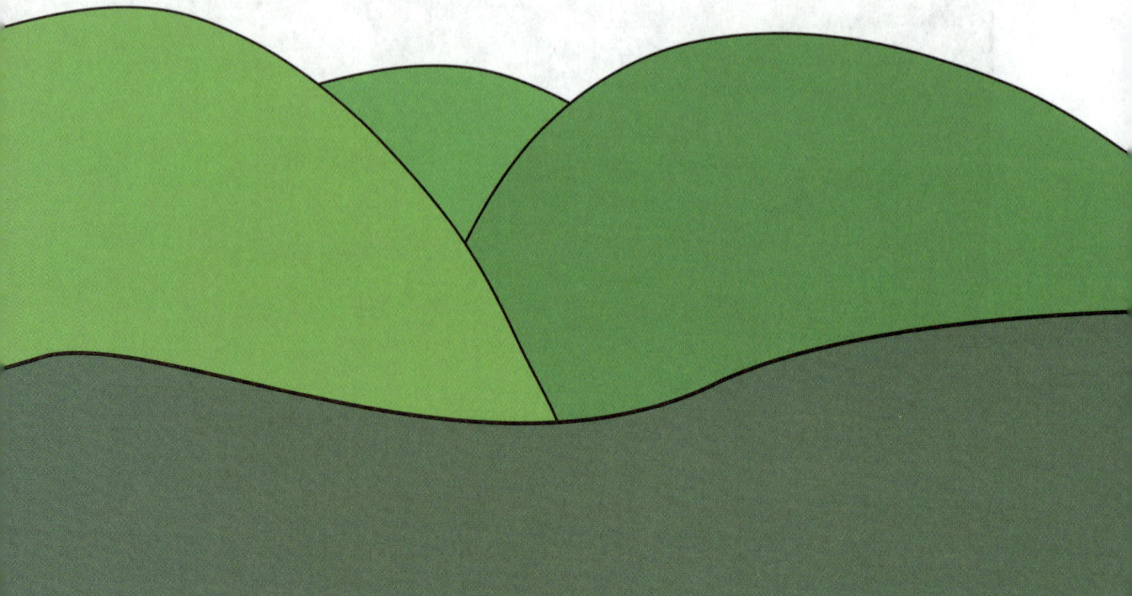

Helping the Bereaved

- Encourage the person to express his/her grief.
- Be available.
- Listen patiently, do not make thoughts more realistic, accept if it is repetitive.
- Do not give advice; be patient.
- Recognize that anger and hostile reactions—including rebelling against God—might be part of the grieving process.
- Do not push the person to share feelings if he/she doesn't want to.
- Help the person stay with pain; go through the pain with him/her.
- Help the person identify and express different feelings.
- Help accept the feelings present as a normal reaction; you may talk about how people grieve in different ways.
- After some time, encourage redirection of the person's focus.
- Help maintain good healthful eating habits.
- Help to rearrange the grieving person's life.

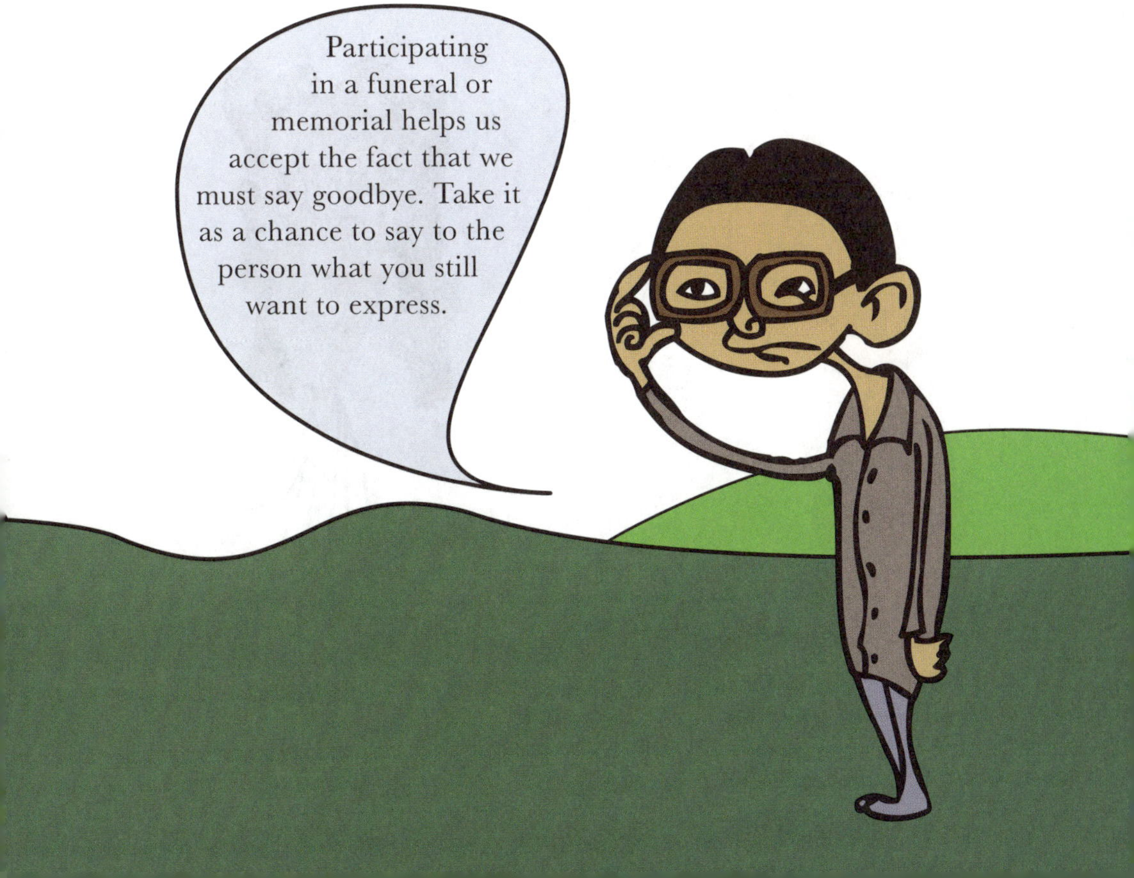
Participating in a funeral or memorial helps us accept the fact that we must say goodbye. Take it as a chance to say to the person what you still want to express.

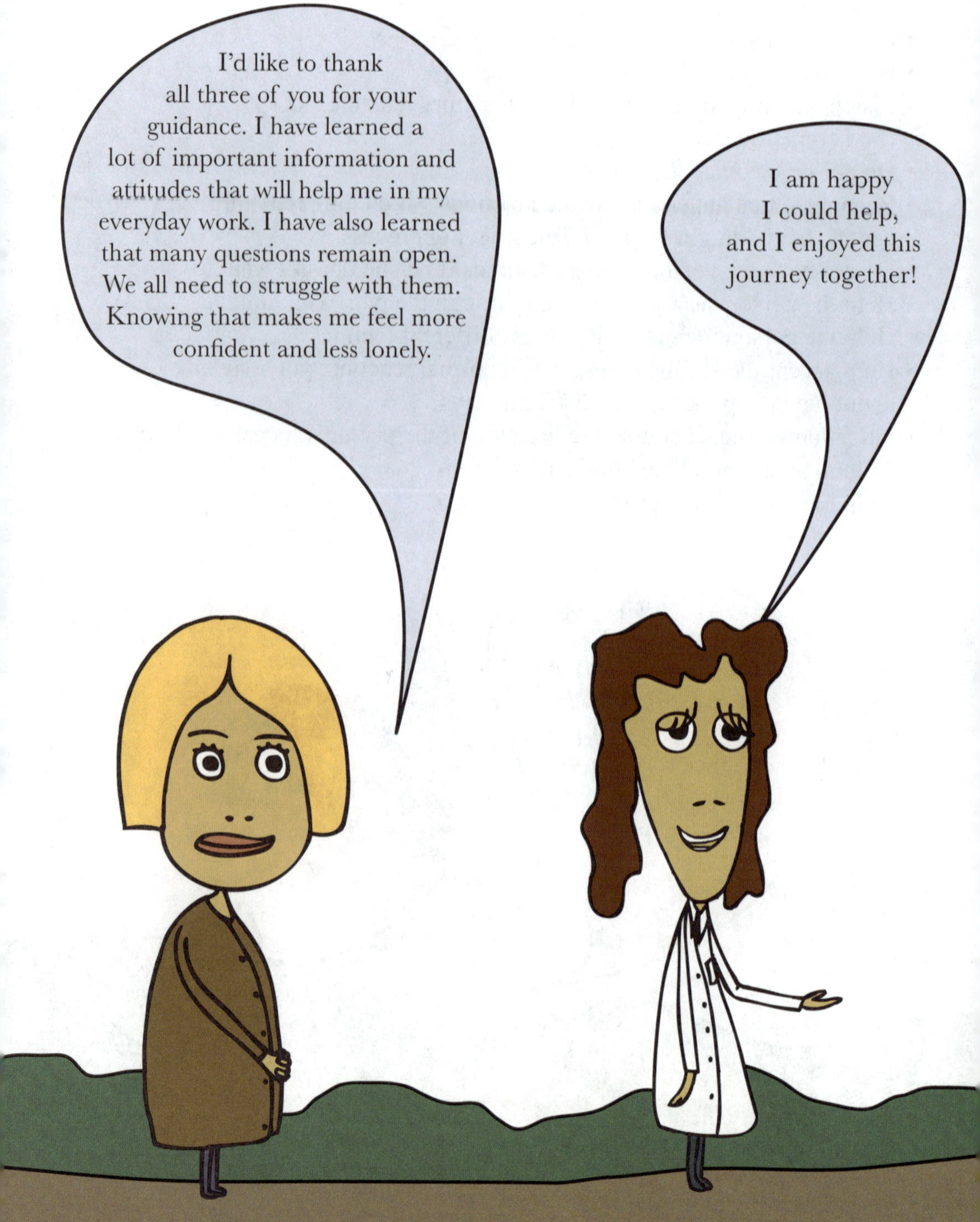
I'd like to thank all three of you for your guidance. I have learned a lot of important information and attitudes that will help me in my everyday work. I have also learned that many questions remain open. We all need to struggle with them. Knowing that makes me feel more confident and less lonely.
I am happy I could help, and I enjoyed this journey together!

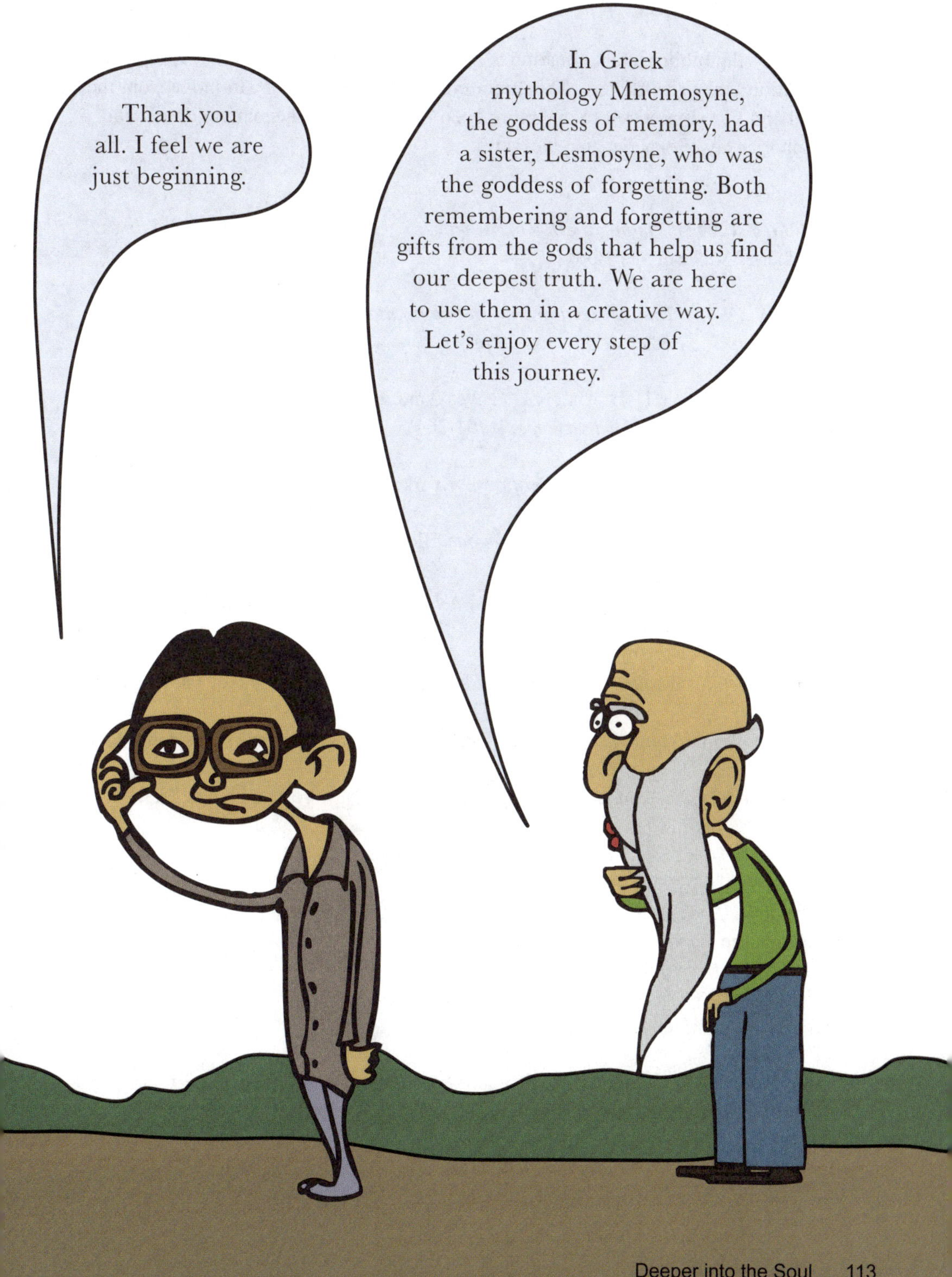
Thank you all. I feel we are just beginning.
In Greek mythology Mnemosyne, the goddess of memory, had a sister, Lesmosyne, who was the goddess of forgetting. Both remembering and forgetting are gifts from the gods that help us find our deepest truth. We are here to use them in a creative way. Let's enjoy every step of this journey.

Bibliography

The following bibliography constitutes the sources and much of the backdrop and inspiration for our work here. This literature also serves as a way to move from the causal and literal mind-set to one more open to the poetic, phenomenological and metaphoric way of experiencing the world.

Avadian, B. (2002). *Finding the Joy in Alzheimer's: Caregivers share the joyful times.* Lancaster, CA: North Star Books.

Barrett, W. (1972). *Time of Need: Forms of imagination in the twentieth century.* Middletown, CT: Wesleyan University Press.

Bateson, G., Jackson, D. D., Haley, J., & Weakland, J. (1956). Toward a Theory of Schizophrenia. *Behavioral Science*. 1(251-264).

Becker, E. (1973). *The Denial of Death*. New York: The Free Press.

Beaufret, J. (2006). *Dialogue with Heidegger*. Bloomington, IN: Indiana University Press.

Bly, R., Hillman, J., & Meade, M. (Ed.) (1992). *The Rag and Bone Shop of the Heart.* New York: HarperCollins Publishers.

Bohm, D. (1980). *Wholeness and the Implicate Order*. London: Routledge & Kegan Paul.

Boss, M. (1971). *Grundriss der Medizin und der Psychologie*. Bern: Verlag Hans Huber.

Boss, M. (1982). *Psychoanalysis and Daseinsanalysis*. New York: Da Capo Press.

Buber, M. (1970). *I and Thou*. New York: Touchstone.

Bugental, E. (2005). *AgeSong: Meditations for Our Later Years.* San Francisco: Elders Academy Press.

Bugental, E. (2007). *Love Fills in the Blanks: Paradoxes of our final years.* Manuscript submitted for publication.

Bugental, J. (1987). *The Art of the Psychotherapist: How to develop the skills that take psychotherapy beyond science*. New York: W. W. Norton & Company, Inc.

Bugental, J. (1999). *Psychotherapy Isn't What You Think: Bringing the psychotherapeutic engagement into the living moment*. Phoenix: Zeig, Tucker & Theisen.

Butler, R. (2002). *Age, Death and Life Review*. In: Doka, K. (Ed.)
Living with grief: Loss in later life. New York: Hospice Foundation of America.

Campbell, J. (Ed.) (1955). *The Mysteries: Papers from the Eranos Yearbooks*.
Princeton: Princeton University Press.

Capra, F. (1975). *The Tao of Physics*. Boston: Shambhala Publications, Inc.

Castleman, M., Naythous, M., & Gallagher-Thompson, D. (1999). *There's Still a Person There: The complete guide to treating and coping with Alzheimer's*. New York: Perigee Trade.

Coelho, P. (1967). *The Alchemist*. San Francisco: Harper and Row.

Coelho, P. (1997). *Manual of the Warrior of Light*. New York: HarperCollins Publishers.

Dalai Lama, H.H. (1998). *The Path to Tranquility: Daily wisdom*.
New York: Penguin Group.

Easwaran, E. (Tr.) (1985). *The Bhagavad Gita*. Tomales, CA: Nilgiri Press.

Easwaran, E. (1996). *Seeing With the Eyes of Love*. Tomales, CA: Nilgiri Press.

Easwaran, E. (Tr.) (1987). *The Upanishads*. Tomales, CA: Nilgiri Press.

Feil, N. (2002). *Validation Breakthrough: Simple techniques for communicating with people with Alzheimer's type dementia*. Baltimore: Health Professions Press.

Feil, N. (2003). *V/F Validation: The Feil Method: How to help disoriented old-old*.
Cleveland: Edward Feil Productions.

Frank, J. (1961). *Persuasion and Healing*. New York: Schocken Books.

Franz, M. (1974). *Shadow and Evil in Fairy Tales*. Boston: Shambhala Publications, Inc.

Foucault, M. (1972). *The Archaeology of Knowledge and the Discourse on Language*.
New York: Pantheon Books.

Foucault, M. (1965). *Madness and Civilization*. New York: Vintage Books.

Foucault, M. (1954). *Mental Illness and Psychology*. Berkeley: University of California Press.

Gadamer, H. (1992). *Truth and Method*. New York: Crossroad Publishing.

Grof, S. & Grof, C. (1980). *Beyond Death: The gates of consciousness.* New York: Thames & Hudson.

Gullette, M. (2004). *Aged by Culture*. Chicago: University of Chicago Press.

Hafiz. (2001). *Drunk on the Wine of the Beloved: Poems of Hafiz.* Boston: Shambhala Publications, Inc.

Hafiz, & Ladinsky, D. (Tr.) (1999). *The Gift: Poems by Hafiz*. New York. Penguin Group.

Heidegger, M. (1962). *Being and Time*. Malden, MA: Blackwell Publishing.

Heidegger, M. (1966). *Discourse on Thinking*. New York: Harper & Row.

Heidegger, M. (1975). *Early Greek Thinking*. San Francisco: Harper & Row.

Heidegger, M. (2006). *Mindfulness.* New York: Continuum International Publishing Group.

Heidegger, M. (1971). *Poetry, Language, Thought*. New York: Harper & Row.

Helminski, K. (Tr.) (1993). *Love Is a Stranger: Selected lyric poetry of Jelaluddin Rumi*. Boston: Shambhala.

Hillman, J. (1989). *A Blue Fire*. New York: HarperCollins Publishers.

Hillman, J. (Ed.) (1980). *Facing the Gods*. Irving, TX: Spring Publications, Inc.

Hillman, J. (1999). *The Force of Character: And the lasting life.* New York: Ballantine Publishing Group.

Hillman, J. (1983). *Healing Fiction*. Woodstock, CT: Spring Publications, Inc.

Hillman, J. (1997). *The Soul's Code: In search of character and calling*. Warner Books.

Hillman, J. (2004). *The Thought of the Heart and the Soul of the World.* Putnam, CT: Spring Publications, Inc.

Hillman, J. (1972). *The Myth of Analysis*. New York: HarperPerennial.

Hillman, J. & Ventura M. (1993). *We've Had a Hundred Years of Psychotherapy—and the World's Getting Worse*. New York: HarperOne.

Hölderlin, F. (1989). *Hölderlins Werke*. Berlin: Aufbau–Verlag.

Hölderlin, F. (2004). *Poems of Friedrich Hölderlin*. San Francisco: Ithuriel's Spear.
Jung, C.G. (1973). *Memories, Dreams, Reflections*. New York: Vintage Books.

Jung, C.G. (1987). *Synchronicity: An acausal connecting principle*.
London: Routledge & Kegan Paul.

Kierkegaard, S. (1986). *Fear and Trembling*. New York: Penguin Classics.

Kleinman, A. (1980). *Patients and Healers in the Context of Culture*.
Berkeley: University of California Press.

Koestenbaum, P. (1971). *The Vitality of Death*. Westport, CT: Greenwood Press.

Krell, D. (1992). *Daimon Life: Heidegger and life-philosophy*.
Bloomington, IN: Indiana University Press.

Kübler-Ross, E. (1969). *On Death and Dying*. New York: MacMillan Publishing Company.

Levine, P. (1997). *Waking the Tiger: Healing trauma*. Berkeley: North Atlantic Books.

Luke, H. (2001). *The Laughter at the Heart of Things*. New York: Parabola Books.

Luke, H. (1987). *Old Age: Journey into Simplicity.* New York: Parabola Books.

May, R. (1983). *The Discovery of Being: Writings in existential psychology*.
New York: W. W. Norton & Company, Inc.

May, R. (1973). *Man's Search for Himself.* New York: Dell Publishing.

Mindell, Amy (1999). *Alternative to Therapy.* Newport, OR: Zero Publication.

Mindell, Amy (1999). *Coma: A Guide for Friends and Helpers*. Portland: Lao Tse Press.

Mindell, Amy (2003). *Metaskills: The Spiritual Art of Therapy* (2nd edition).
Portland: Lao Tse Press.

Mindell, Arnold (2001). *Dreaming While Awake: Techniques for 24-hours lucid dreaming*.
Charlottesville: Hampton Roads.

Mindell, Arnold (2001). *The Dreammaker's Apprentice: Using heightened states of consciousness to interpret dreams*. Charlottesville: Hampton Roads.

Mindell, Arnold (2007). *Earth-based Psychology: Path awareness from the teachings of Don Juan, Richard Feynman, and Lao Tse.* Portland: Lao Tse Press.

Mindell, Arnold (2004). *The Quantum Mind and Healing: How to listen and respond to your body's symptoms*. Charlottesville: Hampton Roads Publishing Company, Inc.

Mindell, Arnold (2000). *Quantum Mind: The edge between psychology and physics.* Portland: Lao Tse Press.

Mindell, Arnold (1995). *Sitting in the Fire*. Portland: Lao Tse Press.

Molloy, W., & Caldwell, P. (2003). *Alzheimer's Disease*. Toronto: Key Porter Books.

Nin, A. (1967). *The Diary of Anais Nin, Volume 2 (1934-1939).* Orlando: Harcourt Brace & Company.

Oliver, M. (2005). *New and Selected Poems: Volume Two.* Boston: Beacon Press.

Oliver, M. (2004). *Why I Wake Early: New poems by Mary Oliver*. Boston: Beacon Press.

Pascal, B. (1995). *Pensées*. New York: Penguin Group.

Peterson, B. (2004). Voices of Alzheimer's. Cambridge: Da Capo Press.

Raia, P., & Koening-Coste, J. (1996). Habilitation Therapy: Realigning the planets. *Alzheimer's Association Massachusetts Newsletter*, 14(N).

Ram Dass (2000). *Still Here: Embracing aging, changing and dying*. New York: Riverhead Books.

Richards. T., & Tomandl, S. (2006). *An Alzheimer's Surprise Party: New sentient communication skills and insights for understanding and relating to people with dementia*. Glenview, IL: Interactive Media.

Rilke, R. (1992). *Letters to a Young Poet*. San Rafael, CA: New World Library.

Rilke, R. (1989). *The Selected Poetry of Rainer Maria Rilke*. New York: Vintage Books.

Rossi, E. (1993). *Psychobiology of Mind-Body Healing: New concepts of therapeutic hypnosis* (2nd edition). New York: W. W. Norton & Company, Inc.

Roszak, T. (1998). *America the Wise: The longevity revolution and the true wealth of nations*. Boston: Houghton Mifflin Company.

Rumi, J. (2001). *Selected Poems of Rumi*. Mineola, NY: Dover Publications.

Schneider, K. (2007). *Existential-Integrative Psychology*. New York: Routledge.

Schneider, K. (2004). *Rediscovery of Awe: Splendor, mystery and the fluid center of life.* St. Paul: Paragon House.

Shabahangi, R.N. (2002). *Faces of Aging*. Warsaw: Elders Academy Press.

Some, M. (1994). *Of Water and the Spirit: Ritual, magic, and initiation in the life of an African Shaman*. New York: Penguin Compass.

Stafford, W. (1977). *The Way It Is: New and selected poems*. Saint Paul: Graywolf Press.

Stafford, W. (1986). *You Must Revise Your Life*. Ann Arbor: The University of Michigan Press.

Steinem, G. (2006). *Doing Sixty and Seventy*. San Francisco: Elders Academy Press.

Suzuki, S. (2002). *Not always so*. New York: HarperCollins Publishers.

Suzuki, S. (2006). *Zen Mind, Beginner's Mind.* Boston: Shambhala Publications, Inc.

Szasz, T. (1970). *The Manufacture of Madness: A comparative study of the inquisition and the mental health movement.* New York: Harper Torchbooks.

Szymkiewicz, B. (2006). *Zranione Stany Świadomości* [Wounded states of consciousness]. Warsaw: Eneteia.

Tarrant, J. (1998). *The Light Inside the Dark: Zen, soul, and the spiritual life.* New York: HarperCollins.

Tart, C. (Ed.) (1990). *Altered States of Consciousness*. New York: Harper and Row.

Tart, C. (2001). *Waking Up: Overcoming the Obstacle to Human Potential*. Backinprint.com.

Thurman, H. (1951). *Deep Is the Hunger.* Richmond, IN: Friends United Press.

Thurman, H. (1953). *Meditations of the Heart*. Boston: Beacon Press.

Tischner, J. (1993). *Mylenie Wedug Wartosci* [Thinking according to values]. Krakow: Znak Publishing House.

Twardowski, J. (1994). *Wiersze* [Poems]. Bialystok: Lyk Publishing Co.

Watzlawick P., Bavelas J. B., & Jackson D. D. (1967). *Pragmatics of Human Communication: A study of interactional patterns, pathologies, and paradoxes*. New York & London: W.W. Norton & Company, Inc.

Whitman, W. (1959). *Leaves of Grass*. The first (1855) edition. New York: Penguin Group.

Wilber, K. (1979). *No Boundary: Eastern and Western approaches to personal growth*. Boston: Shambhala Publications, Inc.

Wiseman, R.W. (2003). *The Therapies of Literature*. Warsaw: Elders Academy Press.

Yalom, I. (1980). *Existential Psychotherapy*. New York: Basic Books.

Zeisel, J., & Raia, P. (2000). Nonpharmacological Treatment for Alzheimer's Disease: A mind-brain approach. *American Journal of Alzheimer's Disease and Other Dementias*. 15(6).

Some Websites

Forgetfulness Care – Practice and Learning

www.agesong.com	Assisted living management company and developer that believes in the value of aging as an important phase in a human being's development and emphasizes honoring our elderly as wisdom keepers in our society.
www.deeperintothesoul.org	Interactive website about new approaches to forgetfulness based on symptoms of forgetfulness being meaningful and important for deepening who we are as human beings.
www.pacificinstitute.org	Mental health and gerontological training and internship programs which try to help in reconceptualizing the idea of aging to the concept of maturing. Pacific Institute would like to reestablish the role of the elder in our societies.

General Information about Alzheimer's and Dementia

www.alz.co.uk	Alzheimer's Disease International (ADI). The umbrella organization of Alzheimer's disease associations around the world.
www.alz.co.uk/help/associations.html	Information about Alzheimer's Societies in the world.
www.alz.org	Alzheimer's Association in the United States of America. Voluntary health organization dedicated to Alzheimer's care, support and research.
www.alz.org/apps/findus.asp	Information about local chapters of Alzheimer's Associations in the United States of America.
www.alzheimers.org.au	Alzheimer's Australia. Organization providing support and advocacy for Australians living with dementia.
www.alzheimer.ca	Alzheimer's Society of Canada. Organization focused on ways to alleviate the consequences of Alzheimer's and related diseases.

www.alzheimers.org.uk	The Alzheimer's Society. Organization that works to improve the quality of life of people affected by dementia, in England, Wales and Northern Ireland
www.alzheimers.org.za	Alzheimer's South Africa. Organization that provides support, education, training, and information on matters pertaining to all forms of dementia.
www.alzfdn.org	Alzheimer's Foundation of America. Organization interested in providing optimal care and services to individuals confronting dementia, and to their caregivers and families.
www.ahaf.org	The American Health Assistance Foundation. Organization that funds research and provides information about Alzheimer's disease.
www.alzbrain.org	Resource containing information for caregivers and professionals of persons with dementia, sponsored by the dementia education & training program.
www.pbs.org/theforgetting	Site containing information about symptoms and the experiences of Alzheimer's disease, hosted by PBS media enterprise.
www.caregiver.org	Family Caregiver Alliance. American organization that addresses the needs of families and friends providing long-term care at home.
www.asaging.org	American Society on Aging. Association that works toward improvement of the quality of life of older adults and their families.

Process Oriented Approach to Symptoms

The following websites include information about process oriented communication with people in altered, remote states of consciousness including dementia and coma. The reader can also find general information about process work and its perspectives on psychological and social issues on these sites.

www.aamindell.net	Arnold and Amy Mindell
www.comacommunication.com	Stan Tomandl and Ann Jacob

www.creativehealing.org	Pierre Morin and Kara Wilde
www.deepdemocracyinstitute.org	Deep Democracy Institute. Organization that provides awareness-based leadership and facilitation trainings.
www.garyreiss.com	Gary Reiss
www.maxfxx.net	Max and Ellen Schupbach
www.tomrichards.com	Tom Richards

Validation Therapy

www.vfvalidation.org	Validation Training Institute. Information about the Validation method, its training and related books.
www.validation-eva.com	European Validation Association. An umbrella organization for companies, individuals or foundations that work with the Validation method.

Eldership Perspective

We list here a few websites that provided us with some insights concerning the concept and practice of Eldership. Far from giving the full spectrum of the sources of inspiration, we would like to present some sites that were subjectively interesting to us and might encourage the reader to do further research.

www.abheritage.ca/eldersvoices	Heritage Community Foundation. History and culture of the Aboriginal people as preserved by elders.
www.eldership.net	Project that aims to foster positive and creative attitudes to the later years of life.
www.easwaran.org	This organization offers instruction and guidance in meditation and allied living skills developed by Eknath Easwaran. Their SETU senior retreats are intended for people of retirement age who have fulfilled responsibilities to family and society and are ready to focus on duty to their highest Self.

www.mosaicvoices.org	Programs that aim at bridging divisions in contemporary communities, including the Way of the Mentor - training in core ideas of mentoring, based largely on the writing of Michael Mead.
www.worldcouncilofelders.org	Organization dedicated to share indigenous wisdom with modern cultures.
www.theelders.org	Organization founded by Nelson Mandela, other prominent elders of our times and supporters of the idea that elders serve an important role in our societies.

other titles by elders academy press

AgeSong: Meditations for Our Later Years

Elizabeth Bugental, Ph.D.

Growing old is not an option. But how we age is a choice. At least we like to think so. *AgeSong* gives us a pleasurable nudge and a little inspiration to take charge of our aging. None of us knows how many years this final life-phase will last, but it's a pretty good bet that it will last at least as long as our adolescence. If we can remember back that far, unlike this life-phase, those teens and early twenties seemed to go on forever and we sure didn't have a plan. Now we're old enough and maybe even wise enough to decide how we'd like to live before we die. And maybe we even have the guts to make the choices we need to make to do it in style.

AgeSong can be taken in small doses to direct our thinking toward the possibilities ahead of us rather than the life we've left behind. It provides us a simple, yet profound, breathing space to take in the richness within our reach that could fill our last days with wonder and gratitude.

Elizabeth Bugental spent her 20s and 30s as a Catholic nun in Los Angeles. She has taught on all levels and was, for over a decade, Chairperson of the Department of Theatre Arts at Immaculate Heart College in Los Angeles. Her second career was as a psychotherapist in the San Francisco Bay Area, in private practice and working jointly with her husband of forty years, James Bugental, noted psychologist and author. Elizabeth holds a doctorate in Speech and Drama from Stanford University and a master's degree from Catholic University of America.

other titles by elders academy press

Doing Sixty and Seventy

Gloria Steinem

Gloria Steinem became a spokesperson for issues about aging quite accidentally after declaring to a reporter on the occasion of her fortieth birthday, "This is what forty looks like. We've been lying for so long, who would know?" Because of this casual comment about her age, she received an avalanche of thanks and support from other women facing age discrimination. This caused her to realize the far reaching dimensions of age oppression.

In her inspiring essay and preface, *Doing Sixty and Seventy*, Steinem shares with both humor and seriousness, her views on age stereotyping, the unexpected liberation that comes with growing older, and defines what she perceives as the fact that women become more radical as they age. The essay also sheds light on the forces that shaped her life and, for readers who have only heard bits and pieces about her, the essay offers a primer on Steinem's bold and logical theories. In the essay, Steinem describes turning fifty as "leaving a much-loved and familiar country" and turning sixty "as arriving at the border of a new one" in which she looked forward to "trading moderation for excess, defiance for openness, and planning for the unknown."

In the Preface, written when Steinem is just past seventy and twelve years after the essay was first published, Steinem explains the development of her precious sense of mortality and time.

Elders Academy Press is proud to have published Ms. Steinem's enlightening and thought-provoking essay—thus allowing it to appear for the first time as an independent volume.

Gloria Steinem remains the United States' most influential, eloquent and revered feminist more than three decades after founding Ms. Magazine. A devoted activist and writer, Steinem continues, as she has for more than thirty-five years, to travel nationally and internationally and speak with a calm voice of reason and articulation about gender, racial, and other civil inequity issues.

other titles by elders academy press

Caregiving from the Heart: Tales of Inspiration

Riki Intner, MA and Roberta Cole, MA

Throughout *Caregiving from the Heart* are stories of true experience. We hear from children, friends, relatives and partners, long distance caregivers and many recipients of care. The shared stories help us to navigate the maze of emotion that can be at once tearful and ebullient, gut wrenching and heartwarming. The stories cover moments large and small and often address elder issues of pressing concern—from depression to loss of mobility and even to last chance romance. We learn that there is no right way to care and that caregiving opens windows on the full range of possibility available to us when we participate in one of the most profound adventures of our lives. The stories speak of agony and surprise—of joy and despair—but most of all, of discovery. *Caregiving from the Heart* is like having a support group in your own home.

Roberta Cole is a communications professional. She has hosted and produced programs for WNBC and WYNY radio as well as WNYC, the flagship station of National Public Radio. She has also taught at New York University and recently moved from New York to Sausalito, California with her husband. Together, they proudly raised one daughter.

Riki Intner is a Marriage and Family Therapist. She lives in San Francisco, California with her husband after raising three children who now have children of their own. She has been in private practice for over twenty years and has also conducted workshops and training sessions at conferences, schools, businesses and community events. She has proudly served on the board of her chapter and district Rotary Clubs. She is a Diplomate in Adlerian Psychology.

other titles by elders academy press

Look for the Moon in the Morning

Leda Sanford

Look for the Moon in the Morning is a collection of inspirational essays written especially for women by Leda Sanford, former editorial director of Get Up & Go!, the magazine for women living anew. The magazine received more than 100,000 requests for a brochure featuring a sampling of these essays - which attests to the widespread appeal of Leda's message. These essays express her philosophy that it's never too late to recreate ourselves, to explore new horizons and to enhance our quality of life.

Leda Sanford is a former New York magazine publishing executive of such magazines as American Home, Bon Appétit, Chief Executive, and Modern Maturity. Her fifteen years with AARP, Age Wave Communications and as editor of The Boomer Report exposed her to extensive research on aging and the aging baby boomer. Leda now devotes her time to writing and as a frequent speaker on preparing ourselves for the "new longevity."

For more information about Leda, please see her website at www.ledasanford.com

other titles by elders academy press

Faces of Aging

Nader Robert Shabahangi, Ph.D.

Faces of Aging is a collection of photographs and essays that address the challenges of aging in a society that is not sympathetic to older people.

The result of this negativity deprives us all from interaction with a very valuable segment of the population.

Older people can provide us with experience, knowledge and friendship if we change or attitude toward them and begin to see them as a resource rather than a liability. History and the humanistic tradition have shown us that when respected and valued older citizens can continue to be productive and creative and can contribute to the quality of life.

Faces of Aging is a tribute to elders and is dedicated to removing the veil from the subject of aging. The book invites us to ask how we can remain conscious of the ways in which we impose our own fears of aging, of death, of the changes that invariably occur as we age, onto the elderly themselves: If we ask ourselves to face our own fears of aging and dying, maybe we can begin to understand how these fears express themselves in our interaction with and attitudes toward the elderly.

Nader received his doctorate from Stanford University researching basic philosophical assumptions underlying present-day psychotherapies. He has worked extensively with elders for more than ten years.